Acknowledgements

When asked to write a new reference book on contraception, I responded "Do we need one?" The answer was "Yes, there is a need for a pocket-size manual." Here it is: a book that is comprehensive but *to the point*, addresses basic concepts but deals with controversy.

This book came to be through the heroic efforts and perseverance of the publishing team, three of whom, in particular, deserve my gratitude: Heidi Harrison for not taking "no" for an answer, Jo Green for typing the manuscript but, above all, Tuan Hô for being my "guardian angel" in developing and seeing the project through, and for having "prophetic" patience.

Preface

Contraception is the pillar of reproductive and sexual health. Access to up-to-date information is the right of men and women seeking health in its wider scope. With on-going developments, the science and practice of contraception have become complex. The aim of this publication is to meet the everyday need of busy practitioners by providing an easy-to-follow reference that will help them guide their patients/clients to make informed choices.

Contraception
Contraception

Ali Kubba MB ChB FRCOG MFFP
Consultant Community Gynaecologist and Honorary
Senior Lecturer
Lambeth Primary Care Trust and Guy's, King's &
St Thomas' School of Medicine
London, UK

M Mosby

MOSBY
An imprint of Elsevier Limited.

© 2005 Elsevier Ltd

The
Publisher's
policy is to use
**paper manufactured
from sustainable forests**

ISBN 0-7234-3361-5

Cataloguing in Publication Data
Catalogue records for this book are available from the US Library of Congress and the British Library.

Note
Medical knowledge is constantly changing. As new information becomes available, changes in treatment, procedures, equipment and the use of drugs become necessary. The editors/authors/contributors and the publishers have taken care to ensure that the information given in this text is accurate and up to date. However, readers are strongly advised to confirm that the information, especially with regard to drug usage, complies with the latest legislation and standards of practice.

Printed in China.

Contents

Abbreviations

BMI	body mass index
CICs	combined injectable contraceptives
COC	combined oral contraceptive
DMPA	depot medroxyprogesterone acetate
EC	emergency contraception
EHC	emergency hormonal contraception
IUD	intrauterine device
IUS	intrauterine system
LAM	lactational amenorrhea method
OTC	over-the-counter
PMS	premenstrual syndrome
POP	progestogen-only pill
STI	sexually transmitted infection
VTE	venous thromboembolism

The contraceptive decision

The principles of contraceptive counselling are encapsulated in the *GATHER* model devised by the Population Information Programme of the Johns Hopkins University (Table 1). This model has been expanded and enhanced for its modern application, as follows:

GREET – Provide privacy and dignity; offer a chaperone; emphasize confidentiality

ASK – Take a sexual history; ask and listen to what the patient wants to discuss, and what her/his past experiences are

TELL – Give spoken and written information about contraceptive choices and healthy lifestyles; discuss mode of action, risks and benefits – be non-directive

HELP – Arrive collaboratively at a decision

EXPLAIN – Teach the contraceptive method (how to use it, what to do if it fails); inform about any future communications with timelines; provide alternative sources of information if required. Discuss nuisance side effects; give clear guidance on what constitutes a serious adverse effect for which the patient has to seek advice.

RETURN – Discuss and advise on follow-up

Contraceptive counselling has to be individualized and backed by written information, always using a language that "gets through".[1–5]

Special needs in different reproductive phases

The following considerations, according to each of the reproductive phases, should be given when counselling and helping patients to make decisions on contraceptive methods.

Table 1. Family planning counselling

Family planning counselling can consist of six parts, described by the word GATHER:

G	**Greet** clients in a friendly and helpful way
A	**Ask** clients about their family planning needs
T	**Tell** clients about available family planning methods
H	**Help** clients decide which method they want
E	**Explain** how to use the method chosen
R	**Return** visits should be planned

Source: Counseling makes a difference. Editors' summary. Family Planing Programs. *Population Reports*. Series J, no. 35, November 1987.

For the teenager:
- Dual protection is important. Condoms provide protection against pregnancy and sexually transmitted infections (STIs), but are poorly used by teenagers. Better outcomes are achieved with a combination of a condom and another contraceptive.
- User-independent methods ensure better compliance.
- Ensure that clients have access to information and support, as required.
- Inform about emergency contraception (see *Emergency contraception*).
- Contraceptives must be chosen to suit a "chaotic" lifestyle.
  During the "career years":
- There is a greater need for effective contraception.
- Consider long-acting methods, or sterilization, if the desired family size has been reached.
  During the post-partum period:
- Contraceptive counselling should ideally be started in the prenatal period.
- Breastfeeding should be encouraged and supported, and a contraceptive plan should be discussed to meet the needs of the lactating mother.
- Discuss sexuality issues to help the woman return to a "normal" function.

- Emergency contraception is not contraindicated even for breastfeeding women.

During the perimenopause:
- Effective contraception is essential.
- Methods with added protection against gynaecological conditions are preferred.
- Fertility decline should be taken into account in choosing the contraceptive method.
- Hormonal methods may ease the menopause transition.
- Any disease risk should be carefully assessed, and the risk/benefit ratio regularly re-evaluated (*see* Appendix 1 for risks in women with intercurrent diseases).

Contraceptive risk-profiling

Practice protocols can be drawn from checklists that are based on broad categories of contraindications to various contraceptives.

For any contraceptive:
- Exclude pregnancy
- Investigate abnormal bleeding
- Ensure informed choice
- Take a medication history
- Record previous surgery
- Record allergies.

For hormonal contraceptives, it should be ascertained that:
- Risk factors for venous thromboembolism include family history, antiphospholipid syndrome, immobilization, age, smoking and obesity.
- Risk factors for arterial disease include age, smoking, diabetes, hypertension, thrombophilias, android obesity and family history of premature coronary artery disease.
- Headache history is taken, with special attention to migraine and especially migraine with atypical aura.
- History of hormone-dependent cancers, such as breast cancer, is documented.
- Any hepatic and gall bladder diseases are reported.

For intrauterine contraceptives:

- Full sexual history should be taken, and sexual health risk-profiling conducted.
- Abnormal uterine anatomy, such as congenital abnormalities or severe cervical stenosis, should be excluded.
- Menstrual problems, such as menorrhagia or dysmenorrhoea, should be enquired about.

Screening history

To include:

- Rubella
- Cervical cytology
- Hepatitis B
- Breast awareness.

Sexual health risk-profiling

This entails the use of demographic, behavioural and clinical features to assess the likelihood that the person may currently have an STI or is at high risk of acquiring one.

Sexual health risk factors include:

- Age under 25
- Recent partner change
- Recent unprotected intercourse
- Two or more partners in the past 12 months
- From a high-prevalence area/population
- History of STI in the patient or partner
- One or more of the following symptoms:
  - Abnormal discharge
  - Intermenstrual bleeding
  - Postcoital bleeding
  - Pain (acute or subacute/dyspareunia)
  - Urinary tract symptoms
  - Sexual violence.

Health professionals need to deal with the patient and their own anxiety/embarrassment or discomfort towards taking a sexual history and conducting an effective consultation in a non-judgemental way. Sexual dysfunction is a pathology that may not be declared by the patient and needs to be positively enquired about. It is important to maintain eye contact and use reflective questions (e.g. "Have I got this right?"). Observation of non-verbal messages and accepting signs of distress from the patient help unravel sexual anxieties and past traumas (*see* Table 2 for a sample of a consultation). Sexual history-taking may also include advice on sexual risk reduction (*see ABC of sexual risk reduction*; Table 3).

Communicating risks

The principles of communicating risks are to express risks in absolute, rather than relative, terms. For example, saying that the venous thromboembolism risk with oral contraception increases from 5 in 100,000 to 15 in 100,000 is more understandable and less alarming to the patient than saying the combined pill triples the risk of venous thromboembolism. Table 4 introduces a currency to express risk. Risk also needs to be put in context of life events and risks taken generally (Table 4). Contraceptive users can deal with uncertainty but need clarity.

All the above processes make up the components of informed choice where a woman voluntarily accepts a method having had her concerns addressed through counselling.

Table 2. A sample consultation
When did you last have sex? Was it with your regular partner? If yes, how long have you been together? If no, did you know your partner? Did he use a condom? Are you using contraception?

Table 3. The ABC of sexual risk reduction		
A	Abstinence	*if not*
B	Be faithful to one partner	*if not*
C	Condoms	

Adherence to instructions and continuation of the contraceptive technique is higher with informed choice. Table 5 shows the factors that influence choice.

Table 4. Putting risks of oral contraceptives into context		
Risk magnitude	**Expect about one adverse event per year:**	**Examples: deaths in the UK per year from:**
10 (1 in 1)	Person	–
9 (1 in 10)	Family	–
8 (1 in 100)	Street	Any cause
7 (1 in 1000)	Village	Any cause, aged 40
6 (1 in 10 000)	Small town	Road accident
5 (1 in 100 000)	Large town	Murder
4 (1 in a million)	City	Oral contraceptives
3 (1 in 10 million)	Province/country	Lightning
2 (1 in 100 million)	Large country	Measles
1 (1 in a billion)	Continent	–
0 (1 in 10 billion)	World	–

Data taken from Calman KC, Royston GHD. Risk language and dialects.
BMJ 1997; **315**: 939–942.

Table 5. What influences choice?		
The health professional's perspective	**Method features**	**User's influences**
Familiarity with a method	Safety of the method	Past experiences
Professional judgement	Efficacy of the method	Information from friends/media
Practice, local and national guidance	Tolerability	Perception of own risk
Evidence-based practice	Ease of Use	Lifestyle/relationship
Cost	Ease of access	Reproductive phase
	Cost if OTC	Expectation and tolerance of side effects
		Cultural acceptability

Evidence-based practice

In assessing the evidence base, one needs to consider the strength of any recommendation and the quality of the evidence (*see* Table 6). Currently, only 30% of our practice is evidence-based, but this situation is changing and the evidence base for reproductive and sexual health is expanding. For useful information, see *Evidence-based medicine websites* in Appendix 3.

The medical eligibility criteria for contraception are summarized in Appendix 1.

Contraceptive prevalence

Figure 1 shows the prevalence of contraceptive methods in the UK. The predominant method for teenagers is the condom, while the pill is the most used method in women in their twenties. Sterilization is the most popular contraceptive technique is women older that 30 years of age, with vasectomy representing 50% of all sterilizations. The prevalence of long-acting contraceptive methods is currently low, but should ideally be increased.

Expressing efficacy[6]

The Pearl Index is the number of failures/pregnancies occurring over 1 year among 100 women using a method. A more comprehensive picture of the efficacy of a method is the Life-Table Analysis model showing cumulative pregnancy rates over a longer period. This is a more realistic assessment of efficacy because contraceptives "get better" with time, as users get more adept at using them. Moreover, those at risk of failure tend to experience failure earlier rather than later.

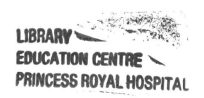

Table 6. Assessing the evidence base*

Strength of recommendations

A   There is good evidence to support the recommendation that the condition be specifically considered in a periodic health examination

B   There is fair evidence to support the recommendation that the condition be specifically considered in a periodic health examination

C   There is poor evidence regarding the inclusion of the condition in the periodic health examination, but recommendations may be made on other grounds

D   There is fair evidence to support the recommendation that the condition be excluded from consideration in a periodic health examination

E   There is good evidence to support the recommendation that the condition be excluded from consideration in a periodic health examination

Quality of evidence

I   Evidence obtained from at least one properly designed randomized controlled trial

II-1   Evidence obtained from well-designed controlled trials without randomization

II-2   Evidence obtained from well-designed cohort of case-control studies, preferably from more than one centre or research group

II-3   Evidence obtained from multiple time series with or without the intervention. Dramatic results in uncontrolled experiments (such as the results of the introduction of penicillin treatment in the 1940s) could also be regarded as this type of evidence.

III   Opinions of respected authorities, based on clinical experience, descriptive studies or reports of expert committees

*Strength of recommendations as suggested by the Canadian Task Force on the Periodic Health Examination.
Reproduced with permission from *Contraception and Office Gynecology: Choices in Reproductive Healthcare*. London: WB Saunders, 1999.

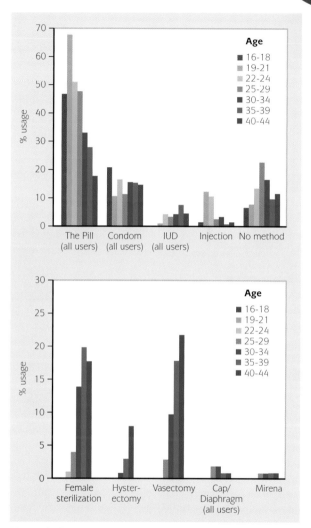

Figure 1. Contraceptive prevalence in the UK. Reproduced with permission from J Brit Menop Soc, September 2003.

The combined pill

The combined pill remains one of the most popular methods of reversible contraception in the world and especially in Western societies. Modern low-dose pills combine high efficacy, convenience, acceptability and an array of non-contraceptive benefits.

Overview

Few drugs have been as thoroughly investigated as the combined oral contraceptive (COC). The pill's contraceptive efficacy and non-contraceptive benefits make it excellent value for money.[7]

Prevalence

The pill is the most popular reversible method in the UK, used by 23% (3.1 million) of contracepting women. The corresponding usage in the US is 17%. Worldwide, 200 million women use the pill.

Mechanism of action

The principal mechanism of action of COCs is inhibition of ovulation through suppression of the hypothalamic pituitary ovarian axis. Endometrial suppression and thickening of cervical mucus are complementary actions. The three actions contribute to the many non-contraceptive benefits of the COC.

Ovarian oestradiol production resumes during the pill-free interval and is suppressed once seven consecutive pills are taken. Prolonging the pill-free interval to 9 or more days may result in enough oestradiol production to trigger a surge in luteinizing hormone and lead to breakthrough ovulation. This is the basis of the missed pill rules.

Pill types

A COC is a combination of a synthetic oestrogen, usually ethinyloestradiol, and a synthetic progestogen (*see* Table 7).

Table 7. Types of combined oral contraceptives by progestogen*

| | Nortestosterone derivatives C-19 progestogens | | | | | Progesterone derivatives C-21 progestogens | Spironolactone analogue |
Levonorgestrel	Norethisterone	Desogestrel	Gestodene	Norgestimate	Cyproterone acetate†	Drasperinone
Ovranette/microgynon 30/microgynon 30ED 30/150	Ovysmen/Brevinor 35/500	Marvelon 30/150	Femodene/ Minulet/ Femodene ED 30/75	Cilest 35/250	Dianette 35/2 mg	Yasmin 30/3 mg
Trinadiol/Logynon/ Logynon ED 30/40/30/50/75/125	Binovum 35/500/1000	Mercilon 20/150	Femodette 20/75			
Eugynon 30 30/250	Trinorum 35/500/750/1000		Triminulet/ Triadene 30/40/30/50/70/100			
Seasonale‡ (extended use for 84 days) 30/150	Norimin 35/1000					
Alesse‡ 20/100	Loestrin 20 20/1000					
	Loestrin 30 30/1500					
	Norinyl-1 50g/1000					

*Where not indicated, values are in μg.
†Dianette (Diane 35) is not licensed for contraception in the UK but is used by many as such.
‡Only licensed in the USA.

§Mestranol (a prodrug of ethinyloestradiol)
Ethinyloestradiol
Progestogen

Safe practice is based on selecting a low-risk user (WHO category 1 or 2; *see* Appendix 1) and prescribing a low-dose pill containing no more than 35 μg ethinyloestradiol. Low-dose pills can contain as little as 15 μg oestrogen. In the UK, only one type of pill containing 50 μg oestrogen is marketed but is rarely used.

Pills can be monophasic, with the same dose of oestrogen and progestogen throughout the menstrual cycle, or multiphasic (biphasic or triphasic), with the dose of oestrogen and/or progestogen changing over the cycle. Multiphasic pills have no specific advantage over monophasic ones. The 21-pill format is popular in the UK, whereby a pill is taken daily for 21 days consecutively, followed by a 7-day pill-free interval, during which a withdrawal bleed occurs. In everyday pills, which are popular in the USA, Australia and South Africa, inactive pills are taken during the 7-day pill-free period, thus making the pill-taking cycle uninterrupted and thereby increasing compliance/adherence.

An extended COC regimen allows the continuous use of a monophasic preparation for three to four menstrual cycles. The prototype pill is Seasonale®, which has recently become available in the USA and comprises 84 pills to be taken daily continuously, followed by 7 pill-free days. Extended COC regimens not only aid adherence and reduce the chances of failure, but also provide women with "period-free" contraception. The high incidence of breakthrough bleeding in the early extended-use cycles is compensated for with amenorrhoea later. A further bonus is a reduction of most menstrual side effects, such as headache, total bleeding time, dysmenorrhoea and premenstrual syndrome (PMS). The causes of breakthrough bleeding are listed in Table 8.

Other variations on the extended-use theme include an everyday-pill scheme where placebo pills are replaced with pills containing low-dose oestrogen (10 µg). This scheme aims to prevent "menstrual migraines". Another preparation has 23 active pills, followed by 5 pill-free days. This shorter period aims to reduce the risk of failure when the pill-free interval is prolonged accidentally.

The medical eligibility criteria for COCs are summarized in Appendix 1.

Attributes

COCs have many attributes, including:
- Effectiveness, convenience and safety

Table 8. Causes of breakthrough bleeding

Organic causes – excluded by examination and tests	User/bioavailability causes
• Cervical bleeding – ectropion, cervicitis, cervical carcinoma • *Chlamydia trachomatis* endometritis/cervicitis • Pregnancy, complications of pregnancy (miscarriage, trophoblastic disease)	• Missing pills • Use of interacting drugs • Vomiting • Severe diarrhoea • Vegetarianism – which may reduce the recycled ethinyloestradiol because of low bowel bacterial flora • Absorption disorders, e.g. coeliac disease (not very likely to cause loss of bioavailability) • Smoking – reduces bioavailability of ethinyloestradiol by 20%

Reproduced with permission from *Contraception and Office Gynecology: Choices in Reproductive Healthcare*. London: WB Saunders, 1999.

- Independence of intercourse
- Rapid return of fertility on discontinuation
- Non-contraceptive benefits:
  - Reduction in ovarian cancer within 1 year of pill taking, reaching 50% after 5 years and 60% after 8 years.[8] This protection lasts up to 15 years after pill discontinuation.[8]
  - Reduction in endometrial cancer by 20% after 1 year and by 50% after 4 years of pill taking.[9] This effect lasts up to15 years after pill discontinuation.[9]
  - Ectopic pregnancy risk lowered by 90%
  - Elimination of dysmenorrhoea, menorrhagia and consequent anaemia
  - 50% reduction in pelvic inflammatory disease
  - 30% reduction in symptomatic endometriosis[10]
  - 50% reduction in benign breast disease
  - At least 30% reduction in colon cancer[11]
  - Small reduction in fibroid risk, although this may primarily apply to high-dose progestogen pills[12]
  - Less PMS

- 50% reduction in benign ovarian cysts[13]
- Improvement in acne with most low-dose pills
- Bone-sparing effect which, in women taking the pill beyond the age of 40, has been shown to reduce the risk of fracture up to the age of 65.

Special uses

For acne and seborrhoea, oestrogen-dominant pills such as Cilest®, Yasmin®, Marvelon® and Femodene® are recommended. Any Progestogen-dominant pill, gestodene or drosperinone-containing pills are used when better control of the menstrual cycle is desirable. For menstrual-associated symptoms, a monophasic preparation is used, preferably in an extended regimen. Yasmin is prescribed for water-retention side effects.

Adverse events

These can be broadly divided into three categories: cardiovascular (arterial and venous) events (*see* Table 9), and hepatic and malignant disease.

Venous thromboembolism

COC thrombogenecity results from a combination of oestrogen-induced changes in coagulation factors and progestogen-dependent smooth muscle relaxation. The risk of venous thromboembolism exists in pill users and disappears quickly after cessation of the pill. While venous thrombosis is not uncommon in women of reproductive age, fatality is low (1%–2% of cases).

While the baseline risk of venous thromboembolism is 5/100,000 women/year, the risks with levonorgestrel pills and desogestrel/gestodene have been reported to be 15/100,000 women/year and 25/100,000 women/year, respectively.[14-20] In pregnant women, this risk is 60/100,000 women/year. Women with risk factors should be excluded from using COCs but can be prescribed any progestogen-only method. Thrombophelia is a risk factor for venous thromboembolism, and the prevalence of hereditary thrombophelias varies from

Table 9. Combined oral contraceptives and the risk of cardiovascular disease*

Condition	Background risk (per year)	Magnitude of COC-associated risk	Overall attribute risk†	Risk in pregnancy	Case fatality
VTE	80/1,000,000	3–6 times	160/1,000,000	600/1,000,000	2%
IS	10/1,000,000	2.5 times	15/1,000,000	80/1,000,000	25%
HS	27/1,000,000	1.5 times	14/1,000,000		30%
AMI < 35	Non-smoker 1/1,000,000 Smoker 8/1,000,000	3–6 times	Non-smoker 3/1,000,000 Smoker 35/1,000,000	100/1,000,000	30%‡
AMI > 35	Non-smoker 10/1,000,000 Smoker 88/1,000,000	3–6 times	Non-smoker 31/1,000,000 Smoker 396/1,000,000		

COC = combined oral contraceptives; VTE = venous thromboembolism; IS = ischaemic stroke; HS = haemorrhagic stroke; AMI = acute myocardial infarction
*Data taken from several studies and models.
†Except where indicated, these figures include women with risk factors.
‡Case fatality is highest in < 25 (36%) compared with > 35 (17%).
Reproduced with permission from Contraception and Office Gynecology: Choices in Reproductive Healthcare. London: WB Saunders, 1999.

0.5% for protein C deficiency to 5% in those with Factor V Leiden mutation.[21] A body mass index (BMI) of over 30 is a moderate risk for thrombosis and a relative contraindication to COCs, while a BMI of over 39 is an absolute contraindication.

Ischaemic stroke

Ischaemic stroke is rare in women of reproductive age. The risk is age-dependent, with a background risk increasing from 2/100,000 at the age of 20 to 20/100,000 at the age of 40. COCs raise the risk by 50%, contributing an extra two cases per 100,000 women in their 20s. Migraine without aura doubles the risk, and migraine with aura increases it four times. Smoking and hypertension are each independent risk factors, which triple the risk of ischaemic stroke.[22,23]

Haemorrhagic stroke

Healthy women under the age of 35, who do not smoke, have no increased risk of haemorrhagic stroke. Over the age of 35, haemorrhagic stroke risk doubles with COC use, triples with smoking and increases 10 times with history of hypertension.[22]

Myocardial Infarction

This is quite rare in young women. Healthy non-smokers under the age of 35 have an excess risk of under 3/million/year. Those over the age of 35, who smoke, have an excess risk of 400/million/year.[24]

Hepatic Disease

The risk of benign and malignant hepatic tumours, both rare events, is higher in pill users.[25] Cholestatic jaundice develops in some users and gall bladder disease risk is increased.[26]

Breast Cancer

Current and ex-pill users over the age of 35 have negligible risk of breast cancer. The pill increases breast cancer risk only in women under the age of 35 who are recent users of oral contraceptives. Excess risk is small (under 10/100,000), does not significantly affect lifetime risk and disappears within 10 years of COC discontinuation.[27] There is no correlation between breast cancer and duration of pill use, and no multiplicative synergy with either a history of benign breast disease or a family history of breast cancer.

A personal history of breast cancer, however, is a contra-indication to the combined pill.

Cervical cancer

Data from a meta-analysis conducted by the International Agency for Research on Cancer indicate an increased risk of cervical neoplasia by oral contraceptives in women at high risk of human papilloma virus infection.[28] This increased risk was not seen in women who used COCs for less than 5 years. The risk increased three-fold at 5 years and four-fold at 10 or more years, and disappeared within 6 years of discontinuation. The findings also suggest that oral contraceptives do not increase the chances of acquisition of human papilloma virus in women who are not at high risk of infection.[28]

The level of increased risk reported in this study may have been exaggerated by factors such as the study methodologies used, the small number of controls and different patterns of pill use in developing countries, where most of the data were obtained. Indeed, the findings from a more recent systematic review indicate smaller relative risks of cervical cancer in women at high risk of human papilloma virus (1.3 and 2.5 for over 5 and 10 years of oral contraceptives use, respectively).[29]

Despite widespread use of oral contraceptives, cervical cancer is now a rare disease in the UK owing to the successful national screening programme. Pill users can protect themselves against cervical cancer by attending regular cervical screening.[30]

Pituitary microadenomas/prolactinomas

Oestrogen stimulates prolactin production in women with pituitary microadenomas/prolactinomas. However, there is no acceleration in the rate of tumour growth. Progestogen-only contraceptives are preferred.

Side effects

Most side effects are transient and lessen with continued use. Oestrogen-dominance side effects require a change to a pill with less oestrogen or more progestogen. Conversely, progestogen-dominance side effects require a change to a pill with more oestrogen or a different progestogen. Table 10 summarizes the side effects and their relationship to the steroid component of COCs.

Counselling points/instruction on use

- The pill can be started up to the 5th day of the menstrual cycle without additional back-up contraception. A start later than day 5 requires back-up contraception for 7 days.[31]
- The pill is contraindicated in breastfeeding mothers but can otherwise be started on day 21 postpartum.
- Missed pill rules – *see* Figure 2 for the steps to take.
- No STI protection: recommend condoms "as well as" pill.
- Follow up at 3 months and then 6–12 monthly to monitor weight and blood pressure.
- No need for pelvic or breast examination before COC initiation unless clinically indicated.
- No other screening tests are required before initiating COCs.
- Discuss aide-memoires to help adherence.
- Discuss the importance of not prolonging the pill-free interval.
- Warn about breakthrough bleeding in the early cycles. In case of breakthrough bleeding lasting more than 6 months, consider the following actions:
  - Use of COC with increased progestogen content. If this fails, consider COC with increased ethinyl-oestradiol content
  - Switch to a different progestogen with high progesterone-receptor affinity
  - Exclude organic and user causes (*see* Table 8)
  - Advise patient to stop smoking.

Table 10. Side effects attributed to the steroid component of combined oral contraceptives

Side effects attributed to oestrogen	Side effects attributed to progestogen
Breast tenderness/tension	"Bloatedness"
Nausea	Seborrhoea and acne
Headaches	(in androgenic susceptible subjects)
Vaginal discharge	Mastalgia
Premenstrual syndrome/	Lassitude/depression
fluid retention	Loss of libido

Reproduced with permission from *Contraception and Office Gynecology: Choices in Reproductive Healthcare*. London: WB Saunders, 1999.

Every time you miss one or more active pills (days 1–21):

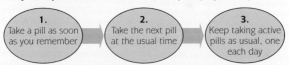

In these special cases, ALSO follow these special rules:

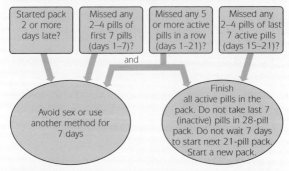

If you miss any of the inactive pills (in a 28-pill pack only):

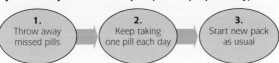

Figure 2. What to do if you miss one or more pills. Source: Johns Hopkins University Bloomberg School of Public Health, Population Information Program. In: World Health Organization. *Selected Practice Recommendations for Contraceptive Use* Geneva: World Health Organization, 2002.

- Reassure about lack of teratogenic effects if the pill is inadvertently taken in early pregnancy.

Tips for safe practice

- Supply written information. Highlight serious adverse events for which the user must seek medical advice (*see* Table 11).
- Emphasize lifestyle risk factors such as smoking.[32]
- There is no added value in taking pill breaks, but a danger of accidental pregnancy.
- Consider drug interaction (*see* Table 12):
  - Women on liver enzyme-inducing drugs should start with a 50-µg pill.[33,34] The dose is titrated upwards depending on cycle control. The pill-free interval should either be omitted or shortened.
  - Women on courses of broad-spectrum antibiotics should use back-up contraception during the course and for 7 days thereafter. Antibiotic courses longer than 2 weeks do not interfere with bioavailability as the bowel bacterial flora recovers.

Post-pill amenorrhoea

This is usually due to one of the known causes of secondary amenorrhoea such as weight-related amenorrhoea, polycystic ovarian syndrome or hyperprolactinaemia. Post-pill amenorrhoea lasting more than 6 months should be investigated as for secondary amenorrhoea.

Yasmin®

Yasmin is a combination of 3 mg drospirenone, the 17-alpha spironolactone derivative, and 30 µg ethinyloestradiol. Drospirenone is closer in action to natural progesterone and has an anti-mineralacorticoid/mild diuretic effect comparable with 25 mg spironolactone. Drospirenone counters the oestrogen-induced fluid retention common to many pills. In some women, fluid retention accounts for side effects such as cyclical weight gain and PMS symptoms.[35] Drospirenone is also an antiandrogen displaying about one-third of the

Table 11. Symptoms following which users of combined oral contraceptives should seek medical advice

Medical advice should be sought following

M Migraine (especially with aura/focal neurological deficit)
U Unilateral pain or swelling in lower limb
C Chest pain or haemoptysis

Reproduced with permission from *Contraception and Office Gynecology: Choices in Reproductive Healthcare*. London: WB Saunders, 1999.

Table 12. Drugs that decrease the efficacy of combined oral contraceptives

Drug group	Examples	Suggested clinical action
Anticonvulsants	Phenytoin Carbamazepine Barbiturates (especially phenobarbitone) Primidone Topiramate	50 µg oestrogen or higher (if breakthrough bleeding), Shorten pill-free interval, extended regimen (e.g. tricycling)
Antibiotics Antituberculous	Rifampicin Rifabutin	Use alternative method, e.g. Depo-Provera
Antifungal	Griseofulvin	Short courses – use additional method, e.g. condoms Long courses – as for anticonvulsants
Antibacterial	Ampicillin, amoxycillin, etc. Tetracylines Broad-spectrum cephalosporins	Short courses – use additional method, e.g. condoms
Wake stimulants	Modafinil	See *Anticonvulsants*
Protease inhibitors	Ritonavir, nelfinavir, nevirapine	See *Anticonvulsants*
Proton-pump inhibitors	Lansoprazole	See *Anticonvulsants*

Table 13. Pharmacological profile of drospirenone and other progestogens

	Progestogenic activity	Glucocorticoid activity	Androgenic activity	Antiandrogenic activity	Antimineralocorticoid activity
Progesterone	+	-	-	(+)	+
Drospirenone	+	-	-	+	+
Levonorgestrel	+	-	(+)	-	-
Gestodene	+	-	(+)	-	(+)
Norgestimate*	+	-	(+)	-	-
Desogestrel†	+	-	(+)	-	-
Dienogest	+	-	-	+	-
Cyproterone acetate	+	(+)	-	+	-

(+) = Negligible at therapeutic dosages
*Principal metabolite: levonorgestrel.
†Active metabolite: 3-keto-desogestrel.
Data taken from Foidart J M, Wuttke W, Bouw G M et al. Eur J Contraceptive and Reproductive Health Care 2000; 5: 124–34.

antiandrogenicity of cyproterone acetate (Table 13). Yasmin is the only licensed contraceptive alternative to dianette/diane 35.[36]

Other potential/theoretical attributes include:
- A possible mild lowering effect on blood pressure.[37,38]
- For women who experience fluid retention symptoms, especially pre-menstrually with or without the pill.[39,40,41]

- Weight neutrality provides an option for women concerned about pill-induced weight gain.[37,38]

Evidence to watch for

- Does weight affect the efficacy of low dose pills? To answer this question we need to study a large number of users. Evidence from small underpowered studies suggests a small reduction in efficacy of about 60%. This translates into a Pearl index of 0.5% versus the quoted index of 0.3%.[42]

- Extended use – a recent review concluded that extending pill-taking up to 3 months was highly acceptable, with only transient cycle control problems. Short-term safety was good but long-term safety was not assessed. Seasonale is the first extended-use product marketed in the USA (Figure 3).[43]

- Quick start – several studies show that starting the pill at any time in a women's cycle is safe as long as pregnancy is excluded. The traditional worry about cycle-control problems is not supported by the evidence.[44]

- COC and STIs[45] – the pill does not seem to increase the risk of acquisition of HIV although a totally conclusive answer awaits further evidence. There does not seem to be an increased risk of acquisition of chlamydia or gonorrhoea in COC users.

- Is low-dose gestodene/desogestrel more "arterial-friendly"? Class B evidence suggests that myocardial infarction and stroke risks may be less in women using these so-called third-generation pills.[46,47,48,49] This is biologically plausible but needs further confirmation and consensus.

- 20-μg oestrogen pills may prove safer especially for "older" users.

- Current quoted venous thromboembolism (VTE) risks are underestimate. All low-dose pills carry a similar VTE risk which my be closer to the risk in pregnancy.

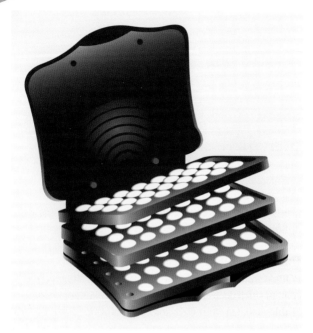

Figure 3. Seasonale. Format and presentation.

The future observed

Dienogest is a new hybrid progestogen of the C19 group but possesses features of the C21 progestogens. 2 mg of this compound are combined with 30 µg ethinyloestradiol in a pill called Valette®, which has the same antiandrogenic profile as Dianette® and offers an alternative in the management of acne.

The first pill with a C21 progestogen (2 mg chlormadinone acetate + 30 µg ethinyloestradiol) is available in some parts of Europe.

The lowest-dose oral preparation is a combination of 15 µg ethinyloestradiol and 60 µg gestodene in a 24-day pill cycle followed by a shortened 4-day pill-free interval.[50]

Progestogen-only pills

Progestogen-only pills (POPs) are reversible, oestrogen-free oral contraceptives. In the UK, the POP is a popular contraceptive choice for breastfeeding mothers.

Overview

The POP like other progestogen-only contraceptives is safe and effective, but causes irregular bleeding in some users. The POP is not a mini version of the combined pill; its use instructions, mechanism of action and safety profile are quite different from those of COCs.

Prevalence

POPs were introduced in the late 1960s and all, except one, contain small doses of either levonorgestrel or norethisterone (Table 14). In the UK, POPs constitute 13% of oral contraceptive use while fewer than 1% of women use this contraceptive option in the USA. Globally, the method is underused, probably because of the preference for long-acting progestogen-only hormonal contraceptives.

Mechanism of action

The most consistent mode of action is thickening of cervical mucus. Ovulation is inhibited in 10% of users. Endometrial and ovarian functions are affected to some degree in about half of users.

Administration

POPs are best taken on the first day of menstruation and daily thereafter without a break. Immediate efficacy is assumed if the POP is started any time within the first 5 days of the cycle.[31] However, in the author's opinion, if compliance is unlikely, the user should be advised to use additional contraceptive precautions if the POP is started after the first 3 days of the cycle.

Table 14. Progestogen-only contraceptives available

Progestogen	Preparation	Progestogen (μg)	No. of pills in pack
Norethisterone	Noriday	350	28
	Micronor	350	28
Levonorgestrel	Microval	30	35
	Neogest	75*	35
	Norgeston	30	35
Ethynodiol diacetate	Femulen	500	28
Desogestrel	Cerazette	75	28

*75 μg norgestrel (= 37.5 μg levonorgestrel).

If the POP is started after the first 5 days of the cycle, back-up contraception is required for 7 days. Postpartum, women whether lactating or not can start the POP on day 21 postpartum without the need for extra precautions or the need to wait for menstruation.

Efficacy

The efficacy of POPs is high during lactation and is critically dependent on compliance. The first-year failure rates for various progestogen-only methods are summarized in Table 15. The ideal use failure rate is under 1%. However, there is an effect of age on compliance, and failure is higher in young users compared with women over the age of 40, in whom the failure rate is 0.3%.[51] The typical failure rate can be as high as 8%.

Attributes

• Medically safe, lowest-dose oral systemic method
• Safe in lactation with minimal transfer of the steroid to the infant (Table 16)[52]

Table 15. First-year failure for different progestogen-only methods

Method	Lowest observed failure rate*	Failure rate in typical users†
No method	85	85
Progestogen-only pills	0.5	2–8
Progestogen-only injectables	0.3	0.3
Norplant	0.04	0.04

*Based on the number of pregnancies occurring among 100 users who use a given method correctly and consistently for 1 year.
†Based on the number of pregnancies in 1 year per 100 typical users of a given method.
Adapted from (1) Hatchet R A, Trussell J, Stewart F et al. editors. Contraceptive Technology, New York: Irvington, 1994; (2) Contraceptive Method Characteristics. Outlook 1992; **10**:1.

Table 16. Estimated steroid intake by fully nursed infants whose mothers use progestogen-only methods

Method (dose)	Daily intake by infant*†
Implants (1st month after insertion)	
Norplant (100 µg/day)	90–100 ng
Implanon (60 µg/day)	75–120 ng
Orals	
Levonorgestrel (30 µg/day)	40–140 ng
Ethynodiol diacetate (500 µg/day)	150–600 ng
Norethisterone (350 µg/day)	100–300 ng
Injectables	
DMPA (150 mg/3 months)	1–13 µg
NET-EN (200 mg/8 weeks)	0.5–2.4 µg

DMPA = depot-medroxyprogesterone acetate;
NET-EN = norethisterone oenanthate

*Estimated from milk concentrations on assumption of daily milk intake 600–800 ml.
Adapted from Collaborative Group on Hormonal Factors in Breast Cancer. Lancet 1996; **347**: 1713–1727.

- Under the woman's control
- Rapid return of fertility on discontinuation
- An alternative when the combined pill causes side effects or is contraindicated
- Unlike the combined pill, efficacy not compromised by broad-spectrum antibiotics
- Reduction of PMS symptoms in some users
- Cardiovascular safety, and therefore popular in women from the age of 35 to the menopause.

Adverse effects/side effects

- Irregular menstrual bleeding in early cycles contributes to the high discontinuation rate: the discontinuation rate for POPs is 60% and half of this is due to bleeding problems.
- POPs have a lower threshold for failure when compliance is poor.
- Functional retention ovarian cysts are seen in 30% of POP users. These are self-limiting and spontaneously reversible, with or without discontinuation.[53]
- There is a small, non-significant increase in risk of breast cancer.[27]
- POPs offer no protection against STIs including HIV.

Counselling points

- Pre-use counselling about irregular bleeding and the small risk of amenorrhoea enhances continued use.
- The user has to be extremely diligent in taking the tablets (*see Missed Pill Rules*).
- Progestogenic side effects such as acne, breast tenderness or headaches can occur.
- Although the overall risk of ectopic gestation is reduced, there are more ectopics in failed POP pregnancies.[54]
- Amenorrhoea is less common but POP is oestrogen-sparing.

Tips for safe practice

- Help the user to incorporate reminders into her pill-taking routine.
- Women weighing over 70 kg may experience higher failure rates and are advised to take two pills a day.[55,56]
- A POP user travelling across time zones can be advised to take a pill at the start of the journey and a repeat dose at the end, or to use physical reminders (e.g. a watch alarm), or leave her watch on the home time as an aide-memoire to taking the next pill.
- The POP is rendered ineffective by liver enzyme-inducing drugs. An alternative method of contraception should be used during the course of such drugs and up to 4 weeks after discontinuation.

Missed pill rules

Any POP except Cerazette® (see page 40 for Cerazette missed pill rules) taken more than 3 hours beyond the regular time is deemed "missed". The forgotten pill should be taken when remembered, and pill-taking routine continued. Precautions should be used from the time a pill is missed until 48 hours after pill-taking is established. If unprotected intercourse takes place anytime during this "window", emergency contraception would be indicated.

Evidence to watch for

- The WHO work on endometrial mechanisms of abnormal bleeding is eagerly awaited.
- The relationship of weight and efficacy of hormonal methods is contentious and requires clarification.

The future observed

Cerazette is a new class of POP that bridges the gap between COCs and the existing POPs. It adds value to and may enhance the popularity of this form of contraception.

Cerazette®

This new POP is in a class of its own. It is oestrogen-free, has a failure rate less than 1% which is independent of the user's age. Cerazette became available in the UK and Europe in 2002. The active ingredient is desogestrel at a dose of 75 μg. Pill-taking rules except for missed pills are similar to the other POPs.[57]

Cerazette has the following special features:

- It is the only anovulant progestogen-only pill. Ovulation is inhibited in 97% of cycles *versus* 60% with a traditional POP. Inhibition of ovulation is a pivotal difference that differentiates this POP from all the others.[58,59]
- Its failure rate is not different from COCs and is consistent among different age groups.[60] Because there is no pill-free interval, correct use may prove to be higher than COCs. The calculated Pearl index in non-breastfeeding mothers is 0.17 for the desogestrel POP *versus* 1.4 for the levonorgestrel POP.
- In bioequivalence, Cerazette is more potent than traditional POPs.
- Being anovulant, Cerazette is not expected to increase the risk of ectopic pregnancy.
- In some users, Cerazette is likely to reduce many of the side effects of menstruation such as dysmenorrhoea.
- Cerazette's licence allows a 12-hour window for a missed pill (similar to COC). When a Cerazette pill is missed back-up contraception is required for 7 days.
- Menstrual irregularity is as common as with other POPs, with prolonged or frequent bleeding more common in the early cycles. However, there is a shift towards infrequent bleeding and amenorrhoea with continued use. Discontinuation rates due to bleeding irregularity are higher than conventional POPs, probably reflecting users' expectations.

- Safety in breastfeeding has been demonstrated.[61] Breastfeeding women experience more amenorrhoea with Cerazette than conventional POPs, a potential advantage in cases of anaemia.
- Progestogenic side effects of breast pain and headaches have been seen in 4 and 7.5 % of users respectively.
- Acne is less frequent with Cerazette compared with a conventional POP.
- Functional ovarian cysts are less likely with Cerazette.

Special indications for Cerazette
- Women who suffer androgenic side effects with traditional POPs
- Women with history of or risk factors for ectopic pregnancy
- Women who had experienced follicular retention ovarian cysts with other POPs
- Women with chronic intercurrent disease where a highly effective contraceptive, entirely under the woman's control, is required and where oestrogen is to be avoided.

Progestogen-only injectables

The market leader is depot medroxyprogesterone acetate (DMPA), or Depo-Provera®, administered 12-weekly. Another progestogen-only injectable is norethisterone oenanthate, or Noristerat®, which is given 8-weekly.

Depot medroxyprogesterone acetate

Overview
DMPA is a cost-effective alternative to female sterilization. It is easy to administer and requires minimal compliance, and the amenorrhea experienced by up to 60% of users at 1 year is seen as a bonus by many. Continuation rates, however, are lower than other long-acting methods and can be improved with careful counselling and ongoing support (Table 17).

Prevalence
The use of Depo-Provera is increasing in the UK and USA with 1% of contraceptors choosing the method. Worldwide, it is used by over 20 million women.

Table 17. Termination at 1 year among users of progestogen-only methods*

Method	All reasons	Bleeding
Levonorgestrel pills 30	60.9	26.0
Norethisterone pills 350	57.7	24.2
DMPA 150	28.8	11.9
NET-EN 200	24.4	1.8
Norplant	22.9	9.5

DMPA = depot-medroxyprogesterone acetate;
NET-EN = norethisterone oenanthate
*Termination rate per 100 women.
Adapted from Philips A, Hahn DW, Klimek S, McGuire J J.
Contraception, 1987; **36**: 181–192.

Mechanism of action

Injectables inhibit ovulation through suppression of the hypothalamic/pituitary/ovarian axis. The complementary mechanisms of action include endometrial suppression and thickening of cervical mucus. Ovarian suppression is associated with hypo-oestrogenism unlike other progestogen only methods, where follicular activity and, therefore, oestrogen production are spared.[62]

Administration

Depo-Provera is a microcrystalline suspension of 150 mg DMPA given by deep intramuscular injection in the thigh or the buttock. The deltoid is an alternative site, especially in overweight women. If given in the first 5 days of the menstrual cycle, no additional contraceptive precautions are required.[31] If given later, back-up contraception should be used for at least 1 week. Hormone levels peak at 3 weeks post-injection, plateau and then drop at the end of the 12-week injection cycle.[31] Women presenting late for their injection have a safety window of at least 7 and up to 14 days. A late injection can therefore still be given as late as 14 weeks without the need for extra precautions.

Efficacy

The ideal and typical use failure rates are the same as no further compliance is required apart from "turning up" for the injection. Failure rates as low as 0.1 per 100 women years have been observed.

Attributes

- Minimal compliance required
- Amenorrhoea – an advantage in case of menorrhagia, anaemia or menstrual symptoms
- Advantages of non-oral methods: no drug interactions, no gastrointestinal side effects, no hepatic first-pass effect
- Ideal for women with bowel disease such as Crohn's disease and ulcerative colitis

- Good choice in sickle cell anaemia as DMPA reduces sickling crisis[63]
- Good choice for women with menstrually induced epilepsy[64]
- A secret contraceptive
- Advantage of an anovulant contraceptive (fewer ectopics, less PMS, less dysmenorrhoea, etc.)
- Over 50% reduction in endometrial cancer risk[65]
- Unaffected by liver metabolism and therefore maybe an option after counselling where liver function is borderline.

Adverse effects/side effects

- Hypo-oestrogeneamia consequent to ovarian suppression is a feature often blamed for a reduction in mineral bone density in long-term users. However, the concern that long-term use may compromise arterial and bone health is not supported by currently available epidemiological data. Bone loss tends to reverse after discontinuation.[66,67,68,69]
  - Women at the extremes of reproductive age (< 18 and > 40 years of age) need careful assessment. Measurement of serum oestradiol is only indicated if there is concern about arterial disease. Bone densitometry is indicated if the user has other risk factors for osteoporosis or is over 45.
  - The UK CSM recently issued guidance that for teenagers, DMPA should only be used as a first line contraceptive if other methods (implants and Cerazette are alternative methods) have been discussed and rejected.
  - Long-term antiretroviral medication reduces bone density. Women receiving antiretrovirals who are on DMPA long term may need closer monitoring of their bone density.
- Reduction in HDL-cholesterol is a disadvantage in "older" women.
- The risk of gall bladder disease is higher.

Table 18. Depot-medroxyprogesterone acetate and reproductive tract cancers (based on WHO studies)

Type of cancer	Relative risk	95% confidence interval
Breast	1.21	0.96–1.52 (ns)
Endometrium	0.21	0.06–0.79 (s)
Ovary	1.07	0.6–1.8 (ns)
Cervix	1.11	0.96–1.29 (ns)

s = statistically significant; ns = not statistically significant

Reproduced with permission from *Contraception and Office Gynecology: Choices in Reproductive Healthcare*. London: WB Saunders, 1999.

- There is no evidence of a statistically significant increased risk of breast cancer (Table 18).[70,71]
- DMPA is not suitable for hypertensive women.
- There is no risk of congenital abnormalities. Masculinization of the external genitalia of a female infant has been reported, but tends to be reversible within weeks.

Counselling points
Informed choice and consent are essential. The following points need to be conveyed to the patient:
- As the injection cannot be removed, the user has to accept the small risk of a side effect that may last the whole duration of the injection cycle.
- Menstrual disruption (breakthrough bleeding and spotting) may occur in the first and second menstrual cycles; 50%–60% of women would be amenorrheac within 1 year and up to 80% at 3 years.
- DMPA serum levels following an injection tend to be high; the user may experience any of the side effects associated with progestogens including mood changes.
- Weight gain tends to occur in a small percentage of users and can be progressive; bloating is a more common reason for complaints of "weight gain".
- Return of fertility is delayed by up to 9 months from the last injection; although almost always transient, post-injection amenorrhoea tends to worry ex-users.

- Injectables offer no protection against STIs including HIV; recent studies suggest a possible association with an increased risk of STIs such as chlamydia.[72]

Postpartum use

DMPA increases the volume, and does not affect the quality, of breast milk. Compared with oral and controlled-release progestogen-only contraceptives, it is likely that more of the steroid is transferred to breast milk. However, observational studies show no long-term impact of DMPA on infant development.

Early postpartum administration of Depo-Provera prolongs lochial bleeding. It is therefore recommended that the first injection is delayed to 6 weeks postpartum to avoid the effect on both the infant and the mother's bleeding pattern. However, initiating the injection at 4 weeks postpartum is allowed in non-breastfeeders. Depo-Provera prolongs lactational amenorrhoea, an advantage in anaemic women.

Tips for safe practice

- Make sure the injection is given intramuscularly as injection into subcutaneous fat can lead to fat necrosis and abscess formation.
- Schedule the next injection at 11 weeks to accommodate those who miss appointments.
- Give a written reminder of the next injection date.
- Long-term users need to be appraised of the theoretical disadvantages of hypo-oestrogenaemia.
- Bone density is reduced in some Depo-Provera users but tends to be mild and to recover on discontinuation.[73] For the majority of users, there is no long-term impact on bone health. Perimenopausal women using Depo-Provera may not have time for bone density recovery but may already have lost the oestrogen-sensitive component of bone.[74] Teenagers under the age of 18 need to be informed of the bone density effect, and given dietary and lifestyle advice to maximize the attainment of peak bone mass.[75] If they remain anxious, an alternative method may be recommended.

- Definition of "long-term" use remains a matter of opinion. Three years of use is a sensible milestone for a discussion on *longer-term* plans.

Management of menstrual disruption

The first-year discontinuation rate for Depo-Provera is up to 30% but, surprisingly, bleeding problems account for fewer than half of discontinuations, perhaps because initial irregular bleeding tends to resolve spontaneously in many users. Pre-use counselling is essential. At least half the users will be amenorrheac at 1 year. Amenorrhoea is a blessing for the majority of women.

If prolonged or frequent bleeding does not resolve, the management strategy is to buy time with an endometrial "stabilizing" treatment until amenorrhoea sets in. Bleeding occurring early in the injection cycle may respond to a course of oestrogen (cyclical or continuous) for two to three cycles. If bleeding tends to occur late in the injection cycle, the next injection can be given early but not earlier than 10 weeks. Mefenamic acid may also be effective. Prolonged abnormal bleeding must be investigated to exclude organic disease.

Norethisterone oenanthate

This injectable is an oily preparation of 200 mg depot norethisterone, which is administered eight-weekly. Global experience is substantial given that there are 2 million users worldwide. The advantages over Depo-Provera include:

- A shorter injection cycle and, therefore, a shorter duration of any endocrine effect or side effects
- Less irregular bleeding and less amenorrhoea
- Higher continuation rates, with under 5% of discontinuations due to bleeding irregularities
- Faster return of fertility.
  The disadvantages compared with Depo-Provera are:
- Liver enzyme-inducing drugs may affect bioavailability/efficacy
- More androgenic
- Currently licensed in the UK for short-term use only.

Evidence to watch for

Research work is ongoing on the bone density impact of Depo-Provera in teenagers and perimenopausal women.

The future observed

For a method that has survived the "boom-and-bust culture" in contraception, the challenge is to develop criteria and protocols for use that will enhance its popularity further.

A 12-weekly subcutaneous version of DMPA (DMPA-SC) at a dose of 104 mg in 0.65 ml is not too far from launch. It provides an option for self-administration.

Monthly combined injectable contraceptives

Overview

Monthly combined injectable contraceptives (CICs) are intramuscular injections combining a long-acting progestogen, which provides the contraceptive effect through ovulation inhibition, and a natural oestrogen to engineer regular bleeds. Owing to the short-acting oestrogen the "bleed" occurs about 2 weeks after the injection, in contrast to pill-withdrawal bleeds.

The two CICs in use are Cyclofem®, or Lunelle®, a combination of 25 mg depot medroxyprogesterone acetate and 5 mg of estradiol cypionate, and Mesigyna®, a combination of 50 mg norethisterone oenanthate and 5 mg estradiol valerate.

Prevalence

Combined injectables have been tested in over 7000 women worldwide. Lunelle was available in the USA, where it had moderate acceptability. Technical and manufacturing reasons have led to a recent withdrawal from the US market.
A combined injectable is expected to be available in the UK in the foreseeable future.

Mechanism of action

Similar to COCs, CICs act through inhibition of ovulation.

Administration

The contraceptive is given by deep intramuscular injection every 30 days (+/- 3 days). The 0.5-ml injection comes preloaded.

Efficacy

The first-year pregnancy/failure rate for Cyclofem/Lunelle is 0.2%, similar to that of COCs.

Attributes

- As a "medium" acting contraceptive, CICs avoid the daily routine of pill-taking thereby reducing default and incorrect use.
- The first-pass effect through the liver is avoided.
- The woman experiences an acceptable bleeding pattern superior to the irregular bleeding of Depo-Provera, but not as good as that of COCs.
- Efficacy may be higher than that of COCs in a typical use situation, as less compliance is required.
- The limited data available on the lipid, carbohydrate and haemostatic balance are reassuring (*see* later). In contrast to COCs, there is no rise in triglycerides.
- Unlike Depo-Provera, CICs are "bone-sparing".
- CICs could be a further choice for teenagers, who would accept injectables but would be concerned about hypo-oestrogenism with Depo-Provera.
- CICs are highly reversible.

Side effects

These are similar to those of COCs. An important point to consider is the need for monthly attendance at a health facility for the injection.

Counselling points

- Irregular or prolonged bleeding may occur in the early injection cycles.
- Amenorrhea is seen in 4% at 1 year.
- CICs are not suitable for self-injection.
- CICs do not confer protection against STIs.
- Weight gain is more likely than with COCs.

Tips for Safe practice

The criteria are no different from the use of other combined hormonal contraceptives.

Evidence that matters

Based on the findings from recent randomized controlled trials, the WHO taskforce on long-acting methods has concluded that, overall, injectable preparations may be safer than oral preparations in not inducing a hypercoagulable state because of reduced synthesis of fibrinogen, and factors VIII and X.[76] However, CICs do slightly reduce the levels of the potent blood coagulation inhibitors, antithrombin III and protein C, and therefore should not be seen as free from the risk of thrombosis. Epidemiological studies are awaited.

The future observed

Subcutaneous CICs are under development and are likely to be suitable for self-injection.[77]

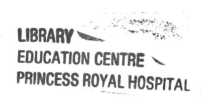

Barrier contraception

Barrier contraceptives physically impede sperm access to the cervix and upper genital tract. They are attractive to many women and men in being non-systemic, totally under the user's control and visible to both partners. Once use is established, no further medical intervention is required.[78]

Condoms

Condoms are the most effective contraceptive barriers, and concomitant spermicide use is no longer recommended.

Male condoms

Male condoms are widely available, and are used worldwide as contraceptives and to prevent STIs including HIV.[79] They can be used alone or for dual protection with another non-barrier contraceptive (*see* Table 19 for the various types of male condom).

Prevalence

In the UK, male condoms are used by over 20% of the population, being second only to the combined pill.

Efficacy

Efficacy is 96%–98% for perfect use, but up to 12% failures are seen in typical use. Efficacy is very user-dependent.[80,81,82]

Attributes/advantages

These include:

- No systemic effects
- Used only when required
- Reduction of risk of STIs, including HIV, chlamydia and pelvic inflammatory disease. *The latex male condom is the gold standard for STI prevention.*

Table 19. Various types of condom

By material	Features
Latex	Low cost, extensive market experience, more allergenic, affected by oil-based lubricants
Natural rubber	Less allergenic than latex, resistant to oil-based lubricants, higher cost
Natural skin (lamb's skin)	Only in USA, sparse data, low allergenicity, thinner than latex, not a barrier against sexually transmitted infections
Polyurethane	Thin, better conduction of heat and sensation, low allergenicity, high cost, possibly higher breakage and slippage rates, odourless, transparent, resistant to oil-based lubricants
By lubricant	
Non-lubricated	May be perceived as "less messy"
Non-spermicidal lubricant	Water-based, preferred
Spermicidal lubricant	No special advantage
By shape	
With teet	Space for ejaculate
Straight shaft	?More sensation
Flared	?More comfortable
Banded latex	Better feel
Loose fitting, bidirectional	EZON (polyurethane) is the only brand – possible lower efficacy
Add-ons	
Coloured, scented, flavoured, fun condoms	e.g. Hip-Hop condoms marketed in the USA in early 2004

- Some protection against human papilloma virus infection
- 50% reduction in cervical neoplasia[83]
- Enhancement of regression of cervical intraepithelial neoplasia by male condoms[84]
- Delay of ejaculation in premature ejaculators
- Easily obtainable.

Side effects/disadvantages

- A coitus-related method needing action during sexual intercourse
- Potential reduction of male or female sexual pleasure
- Not suitable where erectile dysfunction is a problem
- Allergy potentially caused by latex or lubricant
- Breakage and slippage rates as high as 10%.[85]

Counselling points/users' instructions

- Check quality standard of the condom (CE or kite mark).
- Roll the condom on the erect penis before any penile/vaginal contact (the pre-ejaculate has millions of sperms).
- In uncircumcised men the foreskin needs to be retracted first.
- Exit the vagina immediately post-ejaculation whilst securing the condom at the base of the penis.
- Check for breakage and slippage, and ask for emergency contraception if either is observed.
- Avoid oil-based lubricants (*see* Table 20 for information on lubricant use).

Tips for safe practice

- Store condoms away from heat.
- Supply users with written information.
- Demonstrate on "penile model" and teach negotiation skills.[86,87,88]
- Give a realistic picture of efficacy, highlighting reasons for user failures.
- For young people: recommend dual protection with a condom plus another contraceptive.
- Water-based lubricants reduce failures.[89]
- Spermicidal lubrication has no contraceptive or STI-prevention advantage.
- Non-spermicidal lubricants are recommended (*see Evidence that Matters*).

Table 20. Lubricants safe and not safe for use with condoms	
Safe	**Not Safe**
Aci-jel	Aftersun soother; suncream; suntan lotions
Aqueous enemas	Aromatherapy oils; baby oil; bath oil; massage oil
Boots lubricating Jelly	Butter; cream; ice cream; cold cream; low-fat spreads; salad cream
Delfen foam/cream	Canesten
Double Check	Clindamycin cream
Duragel	Clotrimazole
Emko-Foam	Cocoa butter; coconut oil; cooking oil
Glycerine	Cyclogest
K-Y jelly/liquid	Dalacin V cream 2%
Liquid Silk	Ecostatin
Nyspes	Gyno-Daktarin; Gyno-Pevaryl
Nystan pessaries	Hair conditioner; lipstick; vaseline; petroleum jelly; skin products
Ortho-creme; Orthoforms; Ortho-Gynol	Nystan cream
Ovestin cream	Orthogynest
Pevaryl	Sultrin
Replens	
Sensilube	
Staycept pessaries	
Travogyn cream/vaginal tablets	

Female condoms (Femidom®, Reality®)

This is a loose pre-lubricated polyurethane pouch which lines the vagina with the open end left out at the introitus. A soft, free inner ring aids insertion but can be removed once the condom is in place (*see* Figure 4). Alternatively, the erect penis can act as the "inserter". Usage of female condoms is small but not negligible.[90] Femidom is non-spermicidally lubricated.

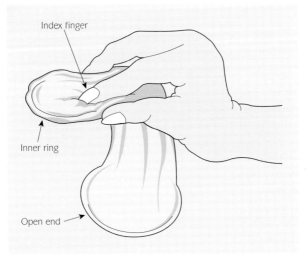

Figure 4. Female condom (Reality®/Femidom®): mode of insertion and structure.

Attributes/advantages
- The attributes and advantages are as for the polyurethane male condom, but with the following significant added advantages:
  - being female-controlled
  - having a perfect use efficacy higher than that of female barriers.[91] This efficacy is probably lower than that of the male condom.
- It can be inserted before intercourse, does not need an erect penis to work and can be used during menses.

Counselling points/users' instructions
- Insert the inner ring high in the vagina, against the cervix.
- Ensure the penis is placed inside, not outside, the condom.
- Concurrent use of the male condom is not recommended as "sticking" can be a problem.
- Supply an information leaflet.
- Advise on emergency contraception.

The future observed
The relatively high cost of the female condom (three times that of the male condom) is a barrier for its use in less developed countries. Re-use after cleansing is therefore an alternative option. Ongoing work suggests that re-use may be safe. Expert guidance from the WHO limits re-use to a maximum of five times, and only with strict adherence to a cleansing and handling protocol.

Spermicides

Nearly all spermicides marketed in developed countries are nonoxynol-9-based (*see* Table 21). Nonoxynol-9, a "detergent", exerts its spermicidal action through destabilizing the spermatozoa cell membrane. When used vaginally, it remains effective for 1 to 2 hours and can be inserted in the vagina up to 1 hour before intercourse. Used alone, spermicides have poor efficacy. Nonoxynol-9 does not protect against gonorrhea and chlamydia.[92]

Evidence that matters
A WHO expert group reported in 2002 that nonoxynol-9 has no contraceptive or STI prevention advantage when used with condoms. Repeated use, defined as more than twice per 24 hours, or prolonged use of nonoxynol-9 alone may increase the risk of HIV acquisition through vaginal epithelial damage.[93] The use of nonoxynol-9 alone is therefore inappropriate and may increase STI risk,[94] in addition to having a failure rate as high as 20%. However, the traditional use of nonoxynol-9 with caps and diaphragms remains an accepted practice. The WHO Medical Eligibility Criteria categorize diaphragm use in women with, or at risk of, HIV as category 3 (*see* Appendix 1 for WHO eligibility criteria).

The future observed
New alternatives to nonoxynol-9 are under development. They fall into two categories: agents that form a protective coating of the vagina (e.g. dextrin-2-sulphate, PRO 2000 Gel) or microbicidal agents (e.g. C31G, Buffer Gel).

Table 21. Spermicide chart[a]

Type of spermicide	Brand name
Gel	*Duragel †Gynol II ‡Conceptrol ‡ Koromex
Cream	*Ortho Cream *Dura Cream
Foam	†Delfen
Pessaries	*Orthoforms ‡Conceptrol inserts (requires 5–15 minutes in vagina to dissolve)
Contraceptive film (less messy, requires 10 minutes in vagina to work)	*C-film ‡Vaginal Contraceptive Film (VCF)
Bio-adhesive	‡Advantage 24

[a]All spermicides are OTC.
*UK only.
†UK and USA.
‡USA only.

Female Barriers

Diaphragms

All diaphragms are made of latex rubber. Traditionally, they are used with a spermicide, which is applied to the saucer-shaped device. A flexible flat or coil-spring ring aids retention between the back of the symphysis pubis and the posterior vaginal fornix. Good manual dexterity is expected, and a user must be able to feel her cervix to verify correct placement.

Prevalence

Fewer than 1% of women using contraception choose diaphragms. However, the diaphragm remains an important choice for women who prefer a non-systemic female-controlled method. It is ideal for "spacers" where efficacy may not be the top priority.

Types

Diaphragms come in sizes of 55–100 mm. Three types are available:

- Flat-spring diaphragms are suitable for nulliparous women with a strong vaginal tone. They fit even with a shallow pubic arch. Pressure on the sides of the diaphragm bends it in a single plane.
- Coil-spring diaphragms have a softer spring and are an option when flat-spring diaphragms may cause discomfort.
- Arcing-spring diaphragms (Ortho All-Flex®; Figure 5) have a firm, double metal spring and are easier to insert as the arcing shape of the diaphragm tends to negotiate the cervix better even when there is some vaginal laxity. Pressure on the sides of the diaphragm bends it in two planes making an arc.

Efficacy

The perfect use efficacy of 92%–96% contrasts with a typical use failure rate as high at 18%.[95]

Attributes/advantages

- Female-controlled use
- Non-systemic
- Potential use as back-up for any other method of contraception
- Permits intercourse during menstruation: menstrual blood is held back
- Reduction in cervical neoplasia risk by at least 50%
- Potential reduction in risk of pelvic inflammatory disease.

Disadvantages

- It is perceived as "messy".
- Can cause latex or spermicide allergy.
- Can cause cystitis symptoms owing to urethral pressure or true urinary tract infection.[96]
- May be expelled especially in women with vaginal prolapse.
- Does not protect against STIs including HIV and herpes.

Counselling points/users' instructions

- Recommend use with spermicides.
- Can be inserted at any time, not necessarily immediately pre-coitus.
- The aim is to fit the largest size diaphragm that is comfortable, ensuring "coverage" of cervix.
- Add spermicide to outer aspect of diaphragm (no need to take diaphragm out) if:
  - 3 hours elapse after insertion
  - the second intercourse takes place beyond 1 hour of first intercourse.
- Leave *in situ* for at least 6 hours after the last intercourse.
- Inspect for holes or misplacement, consider emergency contraception if indicated.
- Replace diaphragm after 12–24 months of use.
- Review the "fit" if the woman loses or gains 7 kg or more in weight.
- Inappropriate for women with high HIV risk.
- The timing for postpartum fitting is at 4–6 weeks.
- Supply written information.
- Warn about oil-based lubricants.
- Schedule a practice period for new users.
- Avoid use if history of toxic shock.
- Advise not to leave in vagina for longer than 30 hours.
- Advise storage away from heat.
- Advise the patient to return if she feels uncomfortable or gets postcoital bleeding.

Cervical caps and other female barriers

The prototype in this group is the Prentif® cavity rim cervical cap (Figure 5). This is a thimble-shaped thick latex device, which comes in sizes of 22, 25, 28 and 31 mm. It is used with a spermicide put in the concavity of the "thimble". Insertion is done by pushing the cap towards the cervix, making it fit on the cervix like a thimble. The cervix therefore needs to be cylindrical and long enough for the cap to fit. At least 10% of women do not have the anatomy to allow the use of this cap.

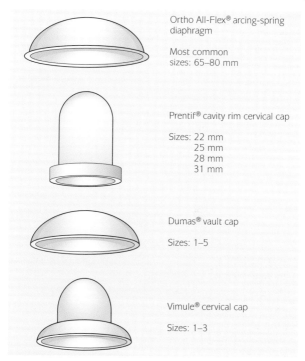

Ortho All-Flex® arcing-spring diaphragm

Most common
sizes: 65–80 mm

Prentif® cavity rim cervical cap

Sizes: 22 mm
      25 mm
      28 mm
      31 mm

Dumas® vault cap

Sizes: 1–5

Vimule® cervical cap

Sizes: 1–3

Figure 5. Cervical barriers.

Advantages/disadvantages and users' instructions

- The advantages/disadvantages and rules of use that apply to diaphragms are valid for all other female barriers. However, fitting cervical caps may require more manual dexterity and urinary tract infections are not a known association.
- Some experts recommend fitting a cervical cap 20 minutes before intercourse to allow the cap to "settle".
- The US FDA recommend a Pap smear test 3 months after cap use, but this is not a rule in the UK.
- Cervical caps do not offer protection against HIV.
- Efficacy is marginally lower than diaphragms.[97]
- A cap is more liable to dislodgement in a woman with a posterior cervix.

- A major advantage of the cervical cap is that it can be left *in situ* for 48 hours.
- The cervical cap is also a better option for women with lax vaginal tone.
- Continuation rates for cervical caps are marginally higher than diaphragms.
- Refitting is still required after pregnancy or a termination of pregnancy because of possible changes in cervical shape and dimensions.
- Anxieties about the risk of toxic shock have not been borne out by experience.

Other caps

Dumas® vault cap

This cap is available in the UK. Made of latex, it is a shallow-domed cap fitting over a short cervix, primarily by suction to the surrounding vagina (Figure 5).

Vimule® cervical cap

This is a latex cap with a thimble dome and a thinner "flared" rim, which allows greater suction (Figure 5).

Lea's Shield®[98]

This cervical cap is made of silicone rubber. Compared with latex, silicone is stronger, tolerant to heat and oil-based lubricants, and less allergenic. It can be left *in situ* for 48 hours. A special feature of the Shield is a one-way valve that allows cervical secretions out, but blocks sperm ascent. The Shield can therefore be used during menses. The thicker posterior section of the Shield fills the posterior fornix and aids retention by sheer bulk.

FemCap®[99]

Femcap combines a sailor's hat shape, silicone rubber durability and a brim that conforms to the vaginal shape (Figure 6). Available in three sizes, it can be left *in situ* for 48 hours but should be kept 8 hours post-intercourse.

Oves® cap

This is a single-use, very thin silicone rubber cervical cap of 0.25-mm thickness (Figure 7). It comes in three sizes (26, 28 and 30 mm), and can be left for up to 72 hours allowing multiple acts of intercourse.

Contraceptive sponges

Protectaid® sponge

An over-the-counter (OTC) product available in a few countries.[100,101] It is made of polyurethane foam combining a mechanical barrier and a spermicidal action. The spermicide is F-5 Gel, which has three agents – sodium cholate, an anti-viral, nonoxynol-9 and benzalkonium chloride – used in smaller doses than in traditional spermicides, thus leading to less vaginal irritation. Efficacy data are extremely limited.

Today® sponge

Recently relaunched in Canada, this sponge contains 1000 μg nonoxynol-9. It can be kept for 24 hours and allows multiple acts of intercourse.

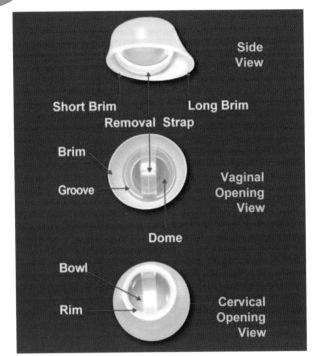

Figure 6. FemCap˙(second generation). Reproduced with permission of FemCap Inc.

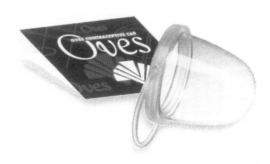

Figure 7. The Oves® contraceptive cap. Source of picture: Mr A Kubba.

Intrauterine devices

The intrauterine device (IUD) remains the "best value for money" reversible contraceptive in existence.

Overview

The prototype ring devices at the turn of the 20th century gave way in the 1960s to the modern inert IUDs, followed swiftly with smaller devices bearing copper. The new generation of devices with high copper content have achieved unsurpassed levels of efficacy and safety.

Prevalence

Globally 150 million women (15% of reproductive-age women) use IUDs. There are spectacular regional differences, with 50% of contraceptors in China using IUDs compared with only 1% in the USA. In the UK, 5% of women use IUDs. Anecdotally, the popularity of IUDs seems to be on the rise.

Mechanism of action[102]

The foreign body reaction created by the IUD encourages phagocytosis and the release of chemical agents toxic to spermatozoa. More importantly, copper itself is a spermicide. The primary mechanism of action is therefore prevention of fertilization through reduction in the sperm population, together with disruption of the tubal ecosystem. Any endometrium-mediated mechanisms are minor and secondary. Even postcoitally, the IUD probably works by degrading the sperm reservoir in the cervical canal and the lower uterine segment, rather than solely through an endometrial effect.

Efficacy

IUDs bearing 300 mm^3 copper or more have an efficacy of around 99%[103] and a lifespan of 5–10 years. The use of IUDs with low copper content is no longer recommended. The market leader, TCu-380A, has a failure rate of 0.6% in year 1 and a cumulative failure rate of 3.4% at 10 years.

IUD removal is recommended when a failure/*in situ* pregnancy occurs as, otherwise, the risks of miscarriage, pre-term delivery and infection are unacceptably high.

Administration

Table 22 is a summary guide to device choice. An IUD can be inserted any time during the menstrual cycle provided that pregnancy is excluded. The optimal "insertion window" is up to day 12 of a 28-day cycle. Postpartum insertion should be delayed until 4 weeks after delivery, and can safely take place up to 6 weeks after delivery in lactating women as the risk of pregnancy up to this time is extremely low.

Post-placental insertion (within 48 hours of delivery) is possible with appropriate training and device selection.[104] However, expulsion rates are higher with such a technique. Post-abortal insertion is also safe and effective,[105] and adverse events are no different from interval IUD insertion. Even insertion after a second trimester abortion may be a viable option although the expulsion rate is higher. Contraindications include pregnancy, distorted uterine cavity, unexplained vaginal bleeding, current or recent (3 months) STI or pelvic inflammatory disease, and trophoblastic disease.[106]

Attributes

- IUDs are effective immediately, and remain effective for years, postcoitally up to 120 hours from intercourse.
- Amongst reversible contraceptives, IUDs are associated with the lowest mortality.
- IUDs allow sexual spontaneity.
- IUDs are associated with at least a 50% reduction in endometrial cancer risk.[107]

Adverse events/side effects

- Menstrual cycle changes include longer, heavier and more painful periods. These account for 15% of discontinuations.

Table 22. Suggested preference order for the use of individual intrauterine devices (IUDs)

Parous women with normal periods

T Safe 380A®
Nova T380®
GyneFix®
ML375®
Flexi-T300®

Nulliparous women with normal periods

GyneFix®
T Safe 380A®
Nova T380®
Flexi-T300®

Women with heavy periods/heavy periods with copper IUD

LNG IUS (Mirena®)

Insertion difficulties encountered

Nova T380®
Flexi-T300®
GyneFix®

Emergency IUD/short-term use in young women

Nova T380®
Flexi-T300®
Nova T200® (while in-date stocks remain)

Reproduced with permission from *J Fam Plann Reprod Health Care* 2002;28:61–68.

- Displacements occur in an average 6% of users. Pelvic ultrasound is the test of choice to confirm correct placement of an IUD. Most displacements occur within 3–6 months of insertion.
- Pelvic inflammatory disease is a risk in the first 20 days post-insertion and tends to be related to pre-existing infections (Figure 8).[108,109] This is a preventable complication through sexual health risk-profiling, STI screening and adherence to an aseptic technique.
- Complete or partial perforation is seen in 1/1000 cases. If detected at insertion, removal of the IUD reduces any associated risks. Later, removal of the IUD may require a hysteroscopic and/or laparoscopic procedure.

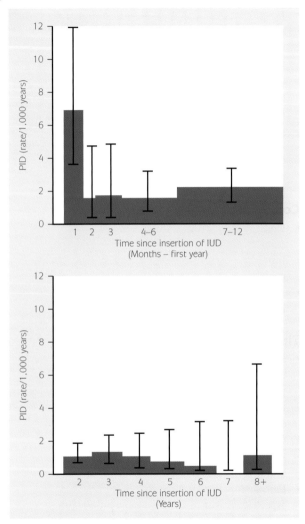

Figure 8. The risk of pelvic inflammatory disease is slightly increased soon after insertion of an intrauterine device. Reproduced with permission from Lancet 1992;339: 785–788.

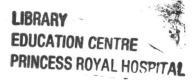

- Ectopic pregnancy – the false apparent excess of ectopics – is due to the high efficacy of the device in preventing intrauterine pregnancies. Among IUD failures, 5–10% are ectopic. However, IUDs reduce the overall rate of ectopic pregnancies from 0.3–0.5% in the general population to 0.02%, a factor of 10–30.[110] Nevertheless, a woman with a history of ectopic pregnancy has a high risk of "recurrence". She should be counselled to use a method that inhibits ovulation, but may use an IUD or intrauterine system (IUS) if she wished.

Counselling points

- Discuss and record counselling on all potential complications.
- Instruct on self-examination of the cervix to confirm the presence of the IUD thread(s).
- Advise to return when symptoms suggest pelvic inflammatory disease or ectopic pregnancy.

Tips for safe practice

- Remember the 7-day rule of not removing an IUD if unprotected intercourse has occurred in the past 7 days, as there is a risk of implantation of a fertilized ovum.
- Consider pain relief for insertion, including the possible use of local/topical anaesthesia.
- Screen for STIs in populations or women at high risk.
- Advise that there is no increased risk of transmitting or acquiring HIV.
- Early follow-up is advised after postpartum, and especially post-placental IUD insertion to exclude expulsion.
- Actinomyces-like organisms are found in cervical smears (Pap tests) in long-term IUD users. To avoid the rare complication of pelvic actinomyces infection, symptomatic women should receive penicillin and consider device removal. Asymptomatic women may

retain or replace their IUDs and should be monitored every 6–12 months.[111]

- An IUD should be removed 1 year post-menopause. A short course of hormone replacement therapy can be given if a difficult removal is anticipated.

- Antibiotic prophylaxis should be considered in emergency fittings where a high risk of STI exists.[112] Routine use of prophylactic antibiotics does not confer benefit.[31]

- An IUD is safe to use in women with valvular heart disease. Insertion and removal should be covered with appropriate antibiotics in women with prosthetic valves and those with history of endocarditis.

Evidence that matters

- IUDs with copper bands such as the TCU-380A and the GyneFix® seem to have a higher efficacy than IUDs with copper wires only. In banded devices, more of the surface area of the copper is "available".

- Previous IUD use does not compromise fertility.[113]

GyneFix®

This is a frameless device with four copper tubes threaded on a polypropylene thread, with two copper tubes crimped at each end (Figure 9).[114] Efficacy is high and the lack of a frame results in lower removal rates for pain, but there is no difference in bleeding or expulsion rates.[115]

The GyneFix has a small insertion diameter and is suitable for women with a tight cervical canal. The fitting technique is different from other devices and needs to be learned. Special indications for the GyneFix include pain with a previous framed device, irregular uterine cavity and expulsion of a previous framed device. Users must be aware of the possibility of a silent expulsion. Most data on the GyneFix comes from studies on parous women. The perforation rate is similar to other IUDs with 12 perforations in 8000 insertions reported in the UK. Removal rates seem to be higher in retroverted uteri.

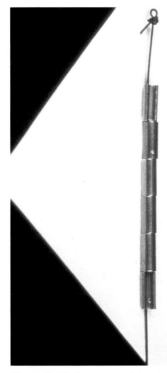

Figure 9. Modern copper intrauterine devices: GyneFix®.
Source of picture: Mr A Kubba.

The future observed

- Further evidence on the extent and mechanism of reduction in endometrial cancer in IUD users would be welcome.
- Long-term randomized controlled trials on efficacy and adverse events are awaited and may suggest that modern IUDs/IUSs have a longer "effective" lifespan.

Intrauterine hormonal contraceptive systems

Mirena®, the levonorgestrel-releasing IUS, is the global market leader (Figure 10). It should not be confused with a progesterone-releasing device, Progestacert®, which is available in the USA. Progestacert has a 1-year lifespan and a high failure rate.

Overview

Mirena fulfils all the criteria of the ideal contraceptive, combining very high efficacy, medical safety and added value in the treatment of idiopathic menorrhagia. In some Western countries, this positive profile has reinvigorated interest in intrauterine contraception. Although IUSs are cost-effective when used long term, the relatively high cost is a barrier to their widespread use in developing countries.

Beyond contraception, Mirena has a therapeutic role in the management of dysmenorrhoea and menorrhagia, and provides opposition at endometrial level to systemic oestradiol stimulation.

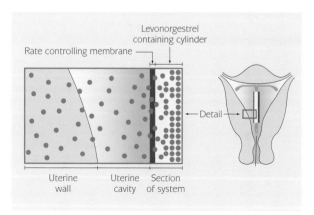

Figure 10. The Mirena® intrauterine system.

Prevalence

Mirena has 2 million users worldwide and is licensed in 74 countries.

Mechanisms of action

The primary action is through a local effect on the endometrium, making the uterine environment hostile to spermatozoa and the endometrium unsuitable for implantation. The secondary mechanisms are thickening of cervical mucus and a variable affect on ovarian function. Between 5% and 50% of menstrual cycles are anovulatory, especially in the first year of Mirena use, owing to the initial higher plasma levels of levonorgestrel (Figure 11).[116] Beyond the first year, most cycles are ovulatory. The amenorrhoea associated with Mirena is due to endometrial suppression and can paradoxically be described as "ovulatory" amenorrhoea.[117]

Mirena contains 52 mg levonorgestrel homogeneously dispersed within the silastic, and covered by a poly-dimethyl-siloxane rate-limiting membrane.[118] It releases 20 μg levonorgestrel/day, although the initial release rate tends to be higher. In the first 3 months of use, plasma levels of levonorgestrel are comparable with those of POPs (this is when side effects tend to occur).[116] The "maintenance" plasma levels of levonorgestrel are one-quarter of the peak progestogen levels in POP users.

Efficacy

There is minimal difference between ideal and typical use failures, with a failure rate of 0.1–0.3% (Figure 12). The 6-year data from a WHO randomized clinical trial show a pregnancy rate of 0.6% and an ectopic rate of 0%.[119] Thus, efficacy is likely to remain high beyond the 5-year Mirena licence.

Interaction with liver enzyme-inducing drugs is presumed to be minimal, although published data lack the power to allow a more robust conclusion.[120]

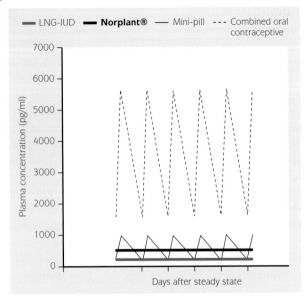

Figure 11. Plasma concentration of levonorgestrel over time after steady state.

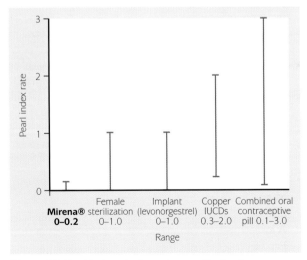

Figure 12. Pearl index rate for various methods of contraception.

Administration

Mirena is 32-mm long and 4.7-mm wide. It has a unique insertion technique which is easy to learn. The basis of the technique is the release of the cross-arms of the device in mid-uterine cavity before advancing the device to its fundal position, thereby minimizing the risk of perforation. The optimal time for inserting Mirena is within the first 5 days of the menstrual cycle. If inserted beyond day 1, back-up contraception should be used for 7 days. Mirena is not effective or suitable for postcoital use. Postpartum insertion is safe from 4 weeks on.

Attributes

- The extremely high long-term efficacy of Mirena makes it the best reversible contraceptive alternative to sterilization.
- With good counselling, the first-year discontinuation rate is as low as 7%.[121] In less developed countries discontinuation is higher owing to intolerance of amenorrhea.
- Mirena has a minimal systemic impact, with a low incidence of progestogenic side effects.
- In contrast to copper IUDs, Mirena reduces menstrual flow and dysmenorrhoea.[122]
- Amenorrhoea enhances continuation, and the first-year amenorrhea rate is 20% rising to 60% with long-term use.
- The number of menstrual cycle bleeding days is reduced from 6 to 1 or 2.
- Iron-deficiency anaemia is prevented.
- The contraceptive effect is immediately reversible on discontinuation.
- Owing to its extremely low ectopic pregnancy rate, Mirena is an option for women with a past history of ectopic pregnancy.[123]
- A lower risk for actinomyces-like organisms is found on Pap smears.
- The risk of pelvic inflammatory disease is possibly reduced.

Therapeutic indications for Mirena

- Mirena is a safe, non-surgical alternative in the management of menorrhagia and is licensed to treat this condition.[124]
  - The impact of Mirena on menorrhagia is substantial, with a 97% reduction in menstrual loss within 1 year.
  - Unlike endometrial ablative techniques, Mirena preserves fertility and provides contraception while in use.
  - Dysmenorrhoea is reduced.[125]
  - Mirena has an efficacy comparable with that of hysterectomy and satisfaction rates similar to those of first and second-generation ablative techniques.[125,126,127]
- Mirena provides progestogen to the endometrium, in opposition to systemic oestrogen in hormone replacement therapy.
  - In peri and early menopausal women who experience erratic bleeding on hormone replacement therapy, Mirena offers a period-free option.
  - The risks of combined hormone replacement therapy, such as breast cancer, are mitigated.[128,129]
  - This therapeutic indication recently received a licence in the UK.
- Other therapeutic indications for Mirena include:
  - Effective treatment for bleeding associated with uterine fibroids[130]
  - Mitigation of tamoxifen-induced endometrial effects[131,132]
  - A role in the management of endometrial hyperplasia without atypia.
  - Reduction of uterine volume in adenomyosis.[133]

Adverse events/side effects

- The most frequent side effect is light bleeding/spotting seen in the first 3 months after Mirena insertion. Women forewarned about this will be prepared and less likely to discontinue.

- Progestogenic side effects may occur during the first 3 to 6 months but tend to disappear with continued use. In long-term users, breast pain, headache and acne occur in 1%, 1% and 1.8% of cases, respectively.
- All the complications associated with IUDs apply to Mirena. Although it may reduce the risk of pelvic inflammatory disease, women at high risk of STIs should be carefully counselled, screened and given sexual health advice.
- Follicular retention ovarian cysts (persistent follicles) occur in up to 10% of Mirena users, compared with 30% with the POP. These are spontaneously reversible.[134]
- Although Mirena can be used in HIV-positive women, it does not offer protection against STIs.
- Continuation rates at 5 years are as high as 65%. Like with other hormonal contraceptives, amenorrhea tends to increase discontinuation rates in some populations. However these are still lower than those of other methods.

Tips for safe practice
Good counselling and comprehensive record-keeping are prerequisites for reducing clinical risk.

Evidence that matters
Research evidence points to apoptosis as the mechanism that reduces menorrhagia and possibly endometrial hyperplasia. Doppler flow studies attempt to elucidate the mechanisms of reduction in menstrual loss. They show a reduction in subendometrial flow at the spiral artery, rather than the uterine artery, level.[135]

The future observed
The next research target is to identify the molecular mechanisms underlying Mirena's actions, which will also allow the expansion its role into the management of endometrial disease.

A Mini Mirena releasing less than 20 μg levonorgestrel/day is in phase II trials.

Fibroplant™ is a frameless levonorgestrel IUS with about half the daily release rate of Mirena (Figure 13). The dose-reduction is supposed to lead to less spotting in the early menstrual cycles.

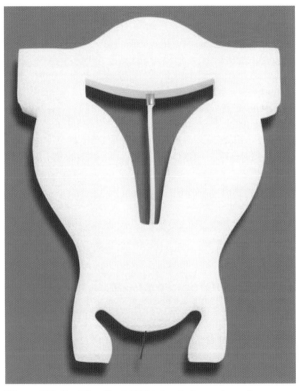

Figure 13. The FibroPlant-LNG intrauterine system after insertion in a uterine model. Courtesy of Dr D Wildemeersch.

Transdermal hormonal contraception

Overview

Evra® is a patch consisting of a three-layer matrix transdermal combined contraceptive system (Figure 14). The middle adhesive matrix layer contains the active hormones (Figure 14b). The matrix is sandwiched between two polyester films, one is beige-coloured to back the adhesive layer (Figure 14c) and the other is the clear release liner (Figure 14a), which is peeled off prior to skin application (Figure 15). An Evra patch releases 20 µg ethinyloestradiol and 150 µg norelgestromin per day for 7 days. The patch is square (4.5 x 4.5 cm) with a total surface area of 20 cm^2.

Prevalence

The Evra patch became available in the UK in mid 2003, having been launched in 2002 in the USA, where there are currently over 1 million patch users.

Mechanisms of action

The mechanisms of action are similar to the COC.

Administration

The Evra patch can be applied to the buttock, the abdomen, the upper outer arm or the torso.[136] The first patch is applied on the first day of menstruation, without need for extra contraceptive cover. Alternatively, a patch can be applied any time in the first 5 days of the menstrual cycle with 7 days of back-up contraception. The patch is replaced with a fresh one once a week on the same "patch-change day". Three weeks of patch use are followed by a patch-free week, after which the next patch cycle starts. Delaying patch change by up to 48 hours does not compromise efficacy, as each patch

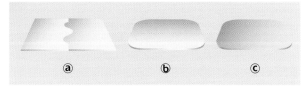

Figure 14. Structure of the EVRA® patch.

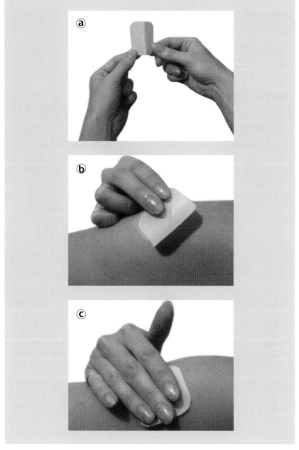

Figure 15. How the EVRA® patch is used: (a) peel; (b) stick; (c) apply. Courtesy of Janssen-Cilag.

continues to deliver adequate ovulation-suppressant hormones
up to 9 days from application. Showering, swimming, baths
and saunas do not appear to affect adhesion.[137]

Efficacy

Evidence from one non-comparative[137] and two randomized
comparative trials[138,139] shows Evra to be as effective as
low-dose COCs, with a failure rate under 1/100 women years.
In contrast to oral methods, the difference between ideal use
and typical use failures is small, reflecting lower propensity
for user error as Evra only requires weekly, rather than daily,
action.[138,139]

Attributes

- Correct use of Evra in teenagers is statistically
  significantly higher than that of oral pills.
  - Correct use of oral pills is age-dependent, with
    incorrect use more prevalent in teenagers.[139]
  - Higher correct use of Evra in teenagers can be
    predicted, but is not proven to reduce failure rates
    in this age group.
  - Typical use failures as high as 8.5% have been
    reported in COC users.[140] Contraceptive efficacy is
    better in cycles of perfect use than those of imperfect
    use.[141,142]
- Efficacy is unlikely to be affected by gastrointestinal
  disturbances or with concurrent use of certain broad-
  spectrum antibiotics such as tetracycline.[143] Although
  back-up contraception is recommended for antibiotics
  other than tetracycline, Evra is likely to be more
  "forgiving" if back-up contraception fails or is not used.
- Like all non-oral methods, the hepatic first-pass effect
  is avoided. Clinical significance, if any, is unknown.
  Concurrent use of liver enzyme-inducing drugs is
  deemed to compromise efficacy, so back-up
  contraception is required.
- 48-hour delayed change window.

- The patch is visible to the user and is therefore "unforgettable".
- The user has 24 hours to take necessary action if the patch is partially or completely detached (*see Counselling points*).

Side effects

- These are similar to those of COCs, except for mastalgia, which is more common in Evra users but tends to resolve with continued use. Interestingly, discontinuation subsequent to mastalgia is similar in the COC and patch groups.[139]
- Patch-site reaction occurs in about 20% of users and tends to resolve spontaneously. It accounts for less than 3% of discontinuation.
- 4.6% of patches detach and need replacement.
- Higher breakthrough bleeding and spotting rate has been reported in the first and second menstrual cycles for the patch (18.3%) *versus* the pill (11.4%). The difference disappears in the third cycle.[139]

Counselling points

- Patch detachment would compromise efficacy. Table 23 summarizes what the user should do with partly or completely detached Evra patches.
  - *Within the last 24 hours*: the partially detached patch should be reapplied; a new patch should be applied to replace a completely detached patch. No additional contraception is required.
  - *Before the last 24 hours*: a new patch should be applied, with the new application day counted as "day 1" (i.e. the new patch-change day). Additional non-hormonal contraception is required for 7 days. Emergency contraception should be considered.
- The above rules also apply if a patch change is delayed more than 48 hours. As this lengthens the patch-free week by 9 or more days, emergency contraception is indicated if unprotected intercourse takes place.

- Any adhesive remaining on the patch site at the end of a 7-day use can be removed with baby oil.

Tips for safe practice

- As Evra transdermal contraceptive has only become available recently further long-term epidemiological studies are needed on aspects of safety and tolerability.
- When disposing a used patch, the user should take care to fold it inwards to avoid environmental contamination with the active hormones.

Evidence that matters

- More efficacy and safety data should become available as use of the Evra patch increases and experience accumulates.
- It is yet to be proven whether transdermal delivery systems have less impact on thrombotic parameters. Limited evidence from transdermal hormone replacement therapy points to a lower impact on such parameters as activated protein C resistance.[144]

Table 23. What to do with partly or completely detached Evra® patches
If detached for <1 day
- Reapply same patch or apply new patch - No additional contraception required
If detached for >1 day (or unknown)
- May not be protected from pregnancy - Apply new patch - Start new cycle   • new day 1 and new patch change day - Additional non-hormonal contraception is required

- A recent Cochrane Review drew three conclusions on the patch: efficacy rates were similar to those of COCs; self-reported compliance was better compared with COCs and breast tenderness was a more common side effect than with COCs.[145]
- Women weighing over 90 kg experience higher failure rates, which are still within the quoted Pearl index of less than 1/100 women years.

The future observed

- An extended patch use regimen (6 weeks of continuous use) has proven to be safe and convenient. The method lends itself to extended use which, in time, may prove to be one of the method's main attractions.
- Teenage users would welcome a range of patch colours and designs, while mature users may be more comfortable with a transparent patch.

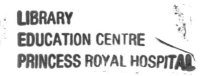

Contraceptive vaginal rings

Overview
Vaginal hormone delivery systems were introduced in the 1970s and have been used successfully in hormone replacement therapy. Progesterone/progestogen-only contraceptive vaginal rings have been seesawing in and out of contraceptive practice with tolerability and safety issues yet to be resolved.[146]

NuvaRing® is the first globally successful combined vaginal contraceptive (Figure 16). It expands the range of new contraceptives that do not require a daily routine. The soft transparent odourless plastic (ethylene vinyl acetate) ring is 54 mm in diameter and 4 mm thick. It releases 15 µg ethinyloestradiol and 120 µg etonorgestrel daily.[147] A steady-state release level is achieved within 3 days of insertion.

Prevalence
The NuvaRing is expected to be available in the UK in 2005. It is already available in the USA, Australia and some European countries. The safety and efficacy data are based on clinical trials of more than 2300 women.

Mechanism of action
The mechanism of action is similar to that of other combined hormonal contraceptives.

Administration
This is a single-cycle contraceptive. The circular ring is inserted by pressing the sides of the circle (Figure 16B) and pushing it into the vagina. Unlike female barrier methods, correct placement is not essential and the relatively small device may be kept in place during intercourse. After 3 weeks of continuous vaginal use, the ring is removed and discarded.

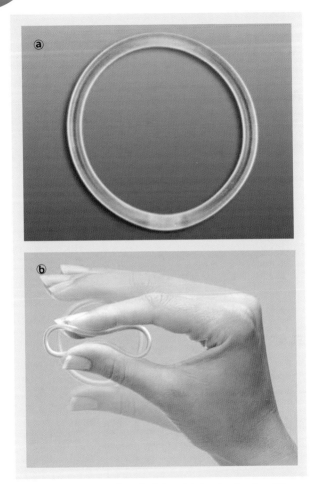

Figure 16. The Nuva® vaginal ring: (a) the circular ring; (b) before insertion into the vagina, the ring is pressed on its sides. Courtesy of Organon.

A 7-day ring-free period is followed by the insertion of a new ring. The ring can be inserted on day 1 of menses, with immediate contraceptive cover, or up to day 5 of the menstrual cycle when 7-day additional contraceptive back-up is required.

Efficacy

The failure rate is under 1/100 women years. Typical use failure (due to non-compliance) is low compared with oral methods.[148]

Attributes

- Compliance-dependent failure is less likely.
- There is no first-pass hepatic effect.
- Efficacy is unlikely to be affected by gastrointestinal conditions.
- Breakthrough bleeding incidence is low.[149,150]
- The bioavailability of the contraceptive hormones is similar to that of COCs, but with maximum hormone levels half those of COCs.[151]
- NuvaRing is moderately oestrogenic, as judged by the levels of sex hormone binding globulin.
- Like all anovulant contraceptives, NuvaRing is likely to reduce menstrual problems and protect against ectopic pregnancies.

Side effects/adverse events

- A comparative study with a standard 30-µg pill shows a lower breakthrough bleeding rate of 5% (mostly spotting) *versus* 10% for the pill.[150]
- The most common side effect is vaginal discharge or inflammation (10.3% of users). Ring expulsion and/or vaginal discomfort were reported in 3.8% and 2.2% of cases, respectively. If expelled, the ring can be rinsed in warm water and re-inserted.
- Reporting of coital discomfort by the male partner is uncommon and is usually tolerated.[147]
- The ring is not suitable for women with vaginal prolapse.
- The ring does not protect against STIs.
- There are no local adverse effects on cervical cytology, or on the integrity of the cervical and vaginal epithelium.

- Progestogenic side effects include headaches (5.8%) and breast tenderness (2.6%). These are no different from other hormonal methods. Overall, discontinuation rate due to side effects is 15.1%, with only about 1% of discontinuation due to cycle-control problems.

Counselling points/tips for safe practice

- If a woman fails to remove the ring after 3 weeks, its hormone reserve gives a safety window of another 7 days and probably longer.
- The use of tampons does not affect the efficacy or the integrity of the ring.
- Vaginal spermicides and antimycotics do not affect efficacy.
- Although intercourse tends not to be affected by the presence of the ring, the couple is allowed to remove the ring for up to 3 hours.
- The ring should be discarded in an environmentally friendly way to reduce environmental contamination by the steroid hormones.

Evidence to watch for

- A recent Cochrane Review failed to find relevant randomized clinical trials.[145]
- Controlled-release delivery systems result in uniform hormone levels, with a single monthly peak, in contrast to COCs with which daily peaks and troughs may contribute to side effects. Further studies in this area would be welcome.

The future observed

- An extended use of the ring for longer than 3 weeks would be an advantage and is being assessed.

Sterilization

Male and female sterilizations constitute the "number one" method of contraception in the developed world. Globally, 18% (187 million) of women of reproductive age depend on sterilization of either sex. In the UK, 50% of sterilizations are vasectomies and the rate of vasectomy prevalence is rising. Sterilization should be seen as a permanent form of contraception. The main advantage is the "one-off investment". The main features of male and female sterilization are listed in the following "fold-out" section.[152]

Female sterilization

Overview

This permanent form of contraception is being challenged by reversible long-acting contraceptives such as Mirena, Implanon and new generation intrauterine devices.

Prevalence

The annual incidence in the UK is around 5/1000.[153] In the UK, 30% of women have been sterilized. However, sterilization rates have been falling from a height of 70,000/year, probably due to a shift to long-acting, reversible methods. In 1999, 47,268 tubal occlusion procedures were performed, 30% fewer operations than the previous decade.

Failure rate

The cumulative rate is 1% over 10 years (Figure 17), three times higher in younger (age < 30 years) people. Fifty per cent of failures are due to technical errors, and 10% are ectopic. Short-term failure is quoted as 1 in 200.

Reversal success[154]

- The reversal success rate is 70% at best, depending of the technique.
- The risk of ectopics is high.

Benefits

- There is at least a 30% reduction in ovarian cancer.[155,156]
- Pelvic inflammatory disease risk may be reduced.

Risks

- Mortality rate is 2–3/100,000 cases.
- Long-term regret has been reported by around 1% of cases.[157]
- There are operative and anaesthetic risks.
- No adverse outcomes have been reported in relation to pain, menstrual dysfunction or menopausal state.

Vasectomy

Overview
- Vasectomy is a minor outpatient procedure.
- It is easier, safer and more effective than female sterilization.
- In the UK, 30% are performed outside hospitals.

Prevalence
- 45 million vasectomies have been performed worldwide.
- Vasectomy is very popular in the UK and the Netherlands, with annual incidence of around 5/1000,[153] and 100,000 sterilizations/year in the UK.
- In 1999, 64,422 vasectomies were performed in the UK.

Failure rate
- The failure rate is 1/1000 cases (1/2000 after "clearance").
- Late failures are possible.[158]
- There is no ectopic risk.

Reversal success
The reversal success rate is 50% at best, inversely related to time from operation.

Benefits
No benefit has been reported.

Risks
- The mortality rate is 1 in 1 million.[159]
- There is no credible evidence of increased risk of prostate or testicular cancer.[160,161]

Female sterilization continued

Counselling points

The following points need to be discussed with the patient:

- Permanency
- Failure and ectopics
- Long-acting reversible alternatives
- Heavy menses if stopping COCs
- The 7-day rule with IUDs
- No need to discontinue oral contraception pre-operatively
- Operative and anaesthetic complications
- Local anaesthesia option.

Tips for safe practice

- There is a need for written consent based on written information.
- Partner consent is not required.
- Ensure that the family is complete (desired family size is achieved), and the patient accepts a non-fertile state in case of a change in relationship or loss of children.
- Ensure that there are no relationship or sexual problems.
- Defer if there are any children under 1 year.
- IUDs can only be removed if preceded by abstinence for 7 days. If in doubt., a pregnancy must be excluded.

Anaesthetic

Sterilization is mostly conducted under general anaesthesia, but local anaesthesia is possible.

Postoperative advice

- Advise rest for 12–24 hours.
- Analgesia for abdominal pain may be needed for up to 3 days.
- Oral contraception should be continued until the end of the current packet.

Postpartum sterilization

This method is popular in the USA and developing countries, but tends to be associated with a higher rate of regret and failures and may require mini-laparotomy

Technique

The most popular technique is tubal occlusion with titanium clips, such as the Filshie Clip. Falope rings and bipolar electrical cautery are still used in some centres.

STI protection

No STI protection has been reported, but there is a possibility of less pelvic inflammatory disease.

Vasectomy continued

Counselling points

These are similar to female sterilization. In addition, mention the following points:

- Postoperative complications of haematoma and sepsis in 2%–3% of cases
- Re-exploration risk about 2/1000
- No increase in sexual dysfunction, cardiovascular disease or quality of orgasm
- Epididymal granuloma formation in fewer than 1% of cases
- Vasectomy is not immediately effective as there is the need to clear the sperm reservoir. This requires an average of 20 ejaculations and two semen analyses (first 12 weeks post-surgery) to confirm clearance.
- In a small minority of men, non-motile sperms persist (< 10,000 non-motile sperm/ml are found at least 7 months post-surgery). In such cases, "special clearance" is given to stop contraception.

Anaesthetic

Local anaesthesia is the norm. General anaesthetic is used if there is an anatomical abnormality, previous surgery or patient preference.

Technique

About 1cm of the vas deferens is cut and removed for histological confirmation. The ends are tied and buried, an operation so-called fascial interposition, which lowers failure rates.[162] Electrical cautery is a less used alternative.

Postoperative advice

- Wear a well-supported jock strap.
- Avoid driving and manual labour for 48 hours.
- Two negative semen analyses are taken 2–4 weeks apart, usually about 2 months from surgery.

STI Protection

No STI protection has been reported.

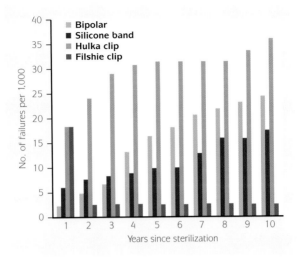

Figure 17. Lifetime cumulative probability of pregnancy among women undergoing tubal sterilization. Data taken from Peterson HB *et al. Am J Obstet Gynecol* 1996;**174**:1161–1170; Filshie GM *et al. Proceedings of the 7th Annual Meeting of the International Society for Gynecologic Endoscopy*; pp 145–158. Bologna: International Proceedings Division, 1998; and Kovacs GT *et al. J Fam Plann Reprod Health Care* 2002;**28**:34–35.

New techniques

- The "no-scalpel" vasectomy technique developed in China is less threatening to men, as it does not involve a cut.[163] Instead, the skin is bluntly punctured. This technique is associated with lower postoperative pain or bleeding, and involves the use of two special instruments (Figure 18).[164]
- A non-incisional hysteroscopic tubal occlusion technique, called Essure, involves tubal cannulation and placement of intrafallopian microinserts (Figure 19).[165] It is performed under local anaesthesia or IV sedation. The Essure device is a small spring-like device made of soft titanium/nickel alloy (Figure 19). Once threaded

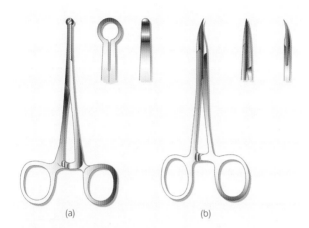

Figure 18. Instrument used for the no-scalpel technique of vasectomy (a) ringed clamp; (b) dissecting forceps. Adapted from No-scalpel Vasectomy: an Illustrated Guide for Surgeons. New York: AVSC, 1992.

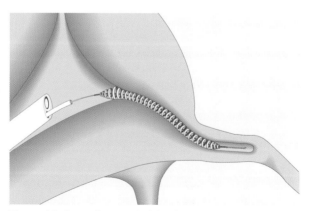

Figure 19. Essure®: a non-incisional approach to fallopian tube sterilization.

into the fallopian tube, a Dacron-like mesh embedded
in the device causes chemical tubal occlusion which is
irreversible. Occlusion is usually complete within
3 months; tubal patency should then be tested.
Long-term efficacy data are awaited. Essure is likely
to be comparable in cost to surgical sterilization.

- In one study, bilateral placement was achieved in
  90% of cases. Short-term follow-up revealed no
  pregnancies.[166]

• The injection of a sclerosing agent, such as Quinacrine
  pellet, *via* an intrauterine vehicle is another minimally
  invasive technique, which has so far been explored in
  small-scale studies.[167,168]

• Transcervical sterilization using thermal (laser or
  diathermy) techniques is also being evaluated.

Evidence that matters

• Failure of both male and female sterilization can occur,
  not only in the first couple of years, but also in later
  years. The 10-year cumulative pregnancy rate for female
  sterilization found in the CREST study was 1.8%.[169]

• Chronic testicular pain seems to be more common post-
  vasectomy. However, as with all subjective outcomes,
  an accurate assessment of risk is not possible.

• Post-tubal occlusion menstrual dysfunction occurs
  primarily owing to age-related incidental pathology,
  against which sterilization does not offer protection.
  Women who have been sterilized are more likely to be
  offered, and more likely to accept, a hysterectomy.

• Reduction in ovarian cancer is an unexpected benefit of
  female sterilization. This effect is substantial and based
  on robust evidence. The underlying mechanism is a
  matter for speculation, but is probably through the
  blockage of the migration and ovarian implantation of
  atypical tubal epithelium.

• The methods of choice for tubal occlusion are the
  Filshie clip or rings. Tubal diathermy should be avoided
  because the risk of subsequent ectopic is higher.

Fertility awareness/natural family planning

Basic information about the fertile phase of the menstrual cycle should be given to all couples to allow them to tailor their contraception for maximum efficacy and/or to plan a pregnancy.[170,171] Menstrual cycle "events" are demonstrated in Figure 20.

Overview

Fertility awareness can be the sole contraceptive method for couples who accept periods of abstinence. For some couples, it may be the only ethically acceptable method. Barrier contraception is an alternative to abstinence during fertile phases.

Prevalence

Fewer than 5% of couples in developed countries, and up to 20% of couples in developing countries, use fertility-awareness as their sole contraceptive. In the UK, the method is taught through a network of recognised trainers. Self-teaching kits and resources are also available.

Principles of fertility awareness

- Ovulation predates the next menses by 14 days.
- Spermatozoa survive in the female genital tract for up to 5 days and, in some extreme cases, up to 7 days.
- The ovum would be available for fertilization for a maximum of 48 hours.
- To predict the fertile phase, a woman has to observe her cycle pattern over several months.
- The fertile phase is thus defined between day 8 and 17 of a regular 28-day menstrual cycle.
- No cycle day is 100% "safe".

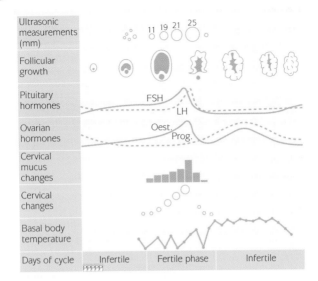

Figure 20. The relationship during the cycle between serial ultrasonic measurements, hormonal control and clinical indicators of fertility. Reproduced with permission from *Contraception and Office Gynecology: Choices in Reproductive Healthcare*. London: WB Saunders, 1999.

Pre-ovulatory events

These include:

- Graafian follicle maturation stimulated by follicle-stimulating hormone released by the anterior pituitary, followed by an increase in follicular oestradiol which induces a surge in luteinizing hormone, leading to follicular rupture and ovum release.[172]

- The parallel events in this oestrogen-dominated phase are endometrial proliferation and increased cervical mucus production. The cervix tends to be high in the vagina. The mid-cycle mucus is copious, clear, thin and stretchy.

Post-ovulation

The corpus luteum releases both oestrogen and progesterone. Progesterone becomes the dominant hormone causing endometrial gland secretion, thickening of cervical mucus, and the closure of the cervix and its relative "descent" in the vagina. Progesterone relaxes smooth muscles and raises the basal body temperature by at least 0.5°C.

If fertilization and implantation do not take place, the negative feedback of oestrogen and progesterone "shut" pituitary gonadotrophins, leading to shedding of the endometrium and the start of another cycle.

Efficacy

This is a method which is intensively dependent on user motivation, compliance and regular menstrual cyclicity.[173] A failure rate of 2% is quoted for couples who adhere strictly to rules and use multiple index methods. The typical use failure rate can be as high as 20%.

Methods of fertility awareness

The calendar method

- Instruct the woman to observe her cycle for 6 months, recording the shortest and longest cycles.
- The beginning of the unsafe/fertile period equals the shortest cycle minus 18. The end of the unsafe/fertile period equals the longest cycle minus 10.
- For a 28–32-day cycle, the unsafe/fertile phase is therefore days 10–22. Unprotected intercourse is allowed up to day 9 and after day 22.
- On its own, this method has poor efficacy.

The temperature method

- Instruct the woman to record the morning temperature in bed, on waking up before any activity.[174]
- The post-ovulation "safe period" starts after 3 consecutive days of a temperature reading at least 0.2°C higher than the preceding day. The couple is

expected to abstain or use of alternative method pre-ovulation.

- The method is best combined with a biological marker such as cervical mucus (this is called combined or mucothermal method).
- "False" temperature readings will result from taking the temperature later in the day, fever, alcohol or stress.

The mucus method (Billings method)

This method is based on cervical changes during the menstrual cycle (Figure 21):

- The user observes changes in cervical secretion, feel (rubbery when "dry"; slippery when "wet") and position relative to the vagina.[175]
- The pre-ovulation "dry" days, with a small volume viscid, turbid mucus, are associated with a firm, closed and low cervix.
- The peri-ovulatory "wet" days start roughly 4 days pre-ovulation with increasing volume, transparency and elasticity of mucus. The cervix is soft and open, and rises in the vagina.
- In post-ovulation, there is a return to the "dry" status.

Intercourse is allowed on dry days within the "safe" window of the calendar method (shortest cycle minus 18) as long as no "wet" days intervene within the "dry" days. The couple should avoid intercourse on successive days in the pre-ovulation phase, as semen may mask the diagnosis of the first "wet" day.[176]

Attributes

- There are minimal long-term costs to the healthcare system and the individual.
- "Unnatural" interventions are avoided.
- The woman is in harmony with her own body and aware of her body rhythm.
- The knowledge gained can be used to achieve a pregnancy when desired.
- Shared responsibility is promoted.

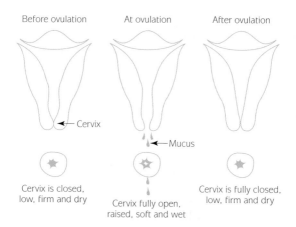

Figure 21. Cervical changes during the cycle.

Disadvantages

- Medical instruction is required initially with a "learning curve" situation.
- Higher efficacy is only seen when intercourse is restricted to the post-ovulatory phase.
- No protection is offered against STIs.
- Fertility awareness is not suitable if the cycle is irregular, such as in adolescence and the perimenopause.
- Fertility awareness requires commitment to a learning phase, self-control and acceptance of periods of abstinence.

Persona®[177]

This portable personal electronic monitor of fertility indices is the size of a pocket diary (Figure 22). The user logs the first day of menses into the monitor, and uses the supplied disposable dipsticks to test her urine for levels of oestrone-3-glucuronide, the main urinary metabolite of oestradiol, and luteinizing hormone to calculate the beginning and the end of the fertile phase, respectively.

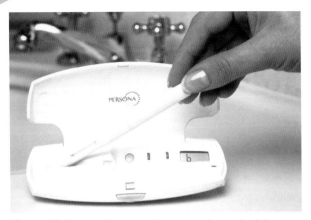

Figure 22. Persona®: a natural contraceptive method that measures luteinizing hormone and can be effective if consistently used in women with regular cycles. (Source of picture: Mr A Kubba.)

The device's "test" threshold for oestrone-3-glucuronide levels corresponds to 5–6 days pre-ovulation (95% of spermatozoa survive 5 days only). The surge in luteinizing hormone is used by the Persona chip to calculate the post-ovulation infertile phase:

- A green light indicates "safe"
- A red light indicates "unsafe"
- A yellow light indicates "test", but abstain/use an alternative method.

An average 16 tests are required in the first cycle, reducing to eight in subsequent cycles, as the device "learns" more about the user's cycle. The failure rate for the method is 6%. The method is not suitable where cycles are outside the 23–35 day range, for women who are 2 months after a pregnancy, are breastfeeding, or use hormonal contraceptive or emergency contraception. It is also not suitable in the presence of hepatic or renal disease.

The Lactational Amenorrhoea Method (LAM)

Exclusive breastfeeding is now recognised as a contraceptive, with an efficacy as high as 98%. The principles of LAM are based on the following three conditions: amenorrhoea; exclusive or near-exclusive breastfeeding (no less than 4-hourly feeding cycle); and being within 6 months post-delivery (Figure 23).[178,179]

In Western countries, the average duration of breastfeeding is 3 months and supplemental feeds are introduced early. This, together with the wide availability of other equally effective contraceptives, underlies the practice of advising back-up contraception (barrier or POP) as early as 6 weeks postpartum.

Evidence that matters

The current 6-month limit for LAM can be applied up to 12 months postpartum, as failure rates remain at an acceptably low level.[180]

The future observed

Although the prospect of women using hand-held user-friendly ultrasound monitors of ovarian activity sounds futuristic, it is possible with current vast technological advances in this area.

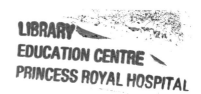

**Ask the mother or advise her to ask herself
these three questions:**

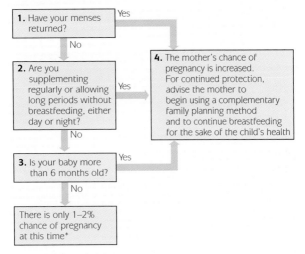

*However, the mother may choose to use a complementary method
at any time

Figure 23. The lactational amenorrhoea method. Reproduced
with permission from *Contraception and Office Gynecology:
Choices in Reproductive Healthcare*. London: WB Saunders,
1999.

Subdermal contraceptive implants

Overview

Subdermal contraceptive implants are progestogen-only methods where the hormone is carried by an inert match-sized polymer. Table 24 shows implants in current use or under development. These implants have a high efficacy, a low user failure rate and high continuation rates.[181] They are seen as alternatives to female sterilization, and are becoming increasingly popular with young people.

- Norplant®, introduced in the 1980s, has a 5-year usage licence and consists of six silastic capsules releasing levonorgestrel. It is available in the USA but was discontinued in the UK in 1999.

- Jadelle®, another levonorgestrel-releasing implant, comprises two silastic rods and has a 5-year usage licence. Although registered in many countries, it is less widely available in practice. Its profile and clinical performance are identical to Norplant but is quicker to insert and remove.[182]

- Implanon® is a single matchstick-sized rod (40 mm long, 2 mm diameter; Figure 24). The device has a 3-year licence and contains 68 mg etonogestrel, which provide a serum level reaching 450 pg/ml initially and stabilizing at 200 pg/ml per day at 3 years. Etonogestrel is the active metabolite of desogestral, which is a low-androgenicity progestogen.[183]

All three implants described are non-biodegradable.

Prevalence

There are currently 11 million Norplant users worldwide, and over 1 million Implanon users.

Table 24. Progestogen implants, presentations and duration of action

Progestogen	Trade name	Presentation	Duration of action
Etonogestrel	Implanon	Single rod	3 years
Levonorgestrel	Jadelle	Two rods	5 years
Levonorgestrel	Norplant	Six capsules	5 years
Nesterone	Elcometrine	Single capsule	6 months
Nesterone	–	Single rod	2 years
Nomegestrol acetate	Uniplant or Surplant	Single rod	1 year

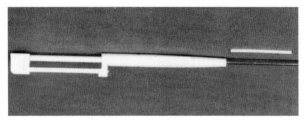

Figure 24. A contraceptive implant device: Implanon®. Source of picture: Mr A Kubba.

Mechanisms of action[184]

All implants inhibit ovulation with low, but constant, levels of progestogen. Ovulation is inhibited mainly through suppression of luteinizing hormone, sparing follicular activity and, therefore, not significantly affecting oestradiol levels. Secondary mechanisms of action include thickening of cervical mucus and endometrial suppression. All implants retain at least half of their progestogen content at the end of their licensed life, which allows a fairly wide margin of error when replacement is due.

Administration

Implants are inserted under local anaesthesia in the superficial subdermal compartment of the inner aspect of the non-dependant upper arm, about 8 cm from the antecubital fossa. The six capsules of Norplant are arranged in a fan shape, opening towards the shoulder. Implanon is inserted in the facial sulcus, between the biceps and triceps muscles. Insertion is effected under local anaesthesia. Being a single rod, Implanon takes an average of 1.1 minutes to insert. Bandaging the insertion site for 24 hours minimizes the risk of bruising. The capsules/rods should be easily palpable, but not normally visible. Insertion is best done in the first week of the cycle.

Removal techniques are easy to learn and depend on the implant type. Difficult removals due to deeply placed implants or implant breakage are only encountered in 1–2% of cases. Adequate training of health professionals in correct insertion techniques minimizes the risk of removal problems.

Efficacy

The ideal-use/typical-use failure range is very narrow, owing to no requirement for compliance. Implants are impressively effective with a failure rate for Norplant of less than 1%. The Implanon research database of over 73,000 cycles and 5,000 women years shows a zero failure rate.[185] Concerns about a reduction in efficacy in overweight women have not been borne out by research.

Attributes of subdermal implants
- Highly effective
- Contraceptive action readily reversible on removal
- Cost-effective if kept for 3 years
- High continuation rates at 85%.

Additional attributes of Implanon
- Easy and quick insertion; easy removal.
- Insertion done with a small amount of local anaesthetic, entailing an "injection" technique. The bevelled tip of

the pre-loaded disposable "injection" cannula is used to puncture the skin. It is then introduced to its full length in the subdermal plane with a tenting movement. A guard/seal is broken and rotated 90°, allowing the cannula to be withdrawn back over the trocar, leaving the Implanon rod *in situ*. Removal is *via* a pop-out technique.

- Suitable for women with acne who wish to use a long-acting progestogen-only contraceptive.
- In contrast to DMPA, weight gain is not such a problem.
- Being an anovulant, Implanon reduces dysmenorrhea.
- Oestrogen-sparing, with no adverse effect on bone mineral density.
- Until further conclusive evidence is available, a woman weighing over 100 kg may wish to consider having her Implanon replaced at 2.5 years, because of a theoretical anxiety about a small reduction in efficacy.

Side effects and disadvantages[186]

- High initial cost, but an implant pays its way because continuation is high.
- Need for removal.
- Ectopic pregnancy rate is lower in implant users than the general population because of the extreme efficacy. However, if an accidental pregnancy occurs, an ectopic should be excluded.
- No protection against STIs.
- The most important side effect is menstrual disruption, especially in the early cycles. With Implanon, the tendency is towards less frequent menstruation and amenorrhoea in at least 20% of cases in the first year (Figure 25).
- Persistent ovarian follicles are seen in Norplant users but not in Implanon users.
- Progestogenic side effects of implants are infrequently reported. They include headaches (20%), weight gain(4–22%), acne/hair problems (3–22%) and mood changes (1–9%).

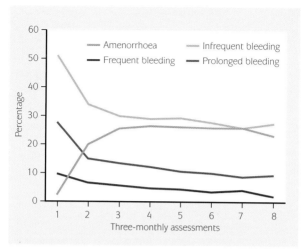

Figure 25. Bleeding patterns with Implanon®.

Counselling points

- Warn about insertion and removal complications, including < 1% risk of infection at insertion site and the possibility of difficult removals (prolonged removals, removals done in more than one sitting and occasionally broken rods).
- Careful counselling about menstrual disruption should stress that any abnormal bleeding tends to be light and reduces with time. There is a net decrease in blood loss in implant users with a concomitant improvement in the haematocrit.
- With Implanon, prolonged or frequent bleeding is seen in about 18% of users but amenorrhoea in 20%–30% of users at 1 year.
- 10–30% of implant users experience progestogenic side effects including acne, mood changes, headaches and mastalgia. These tend to be less with Implanon.
- Implants are ineffective when liver enzyme-inducing drugs are used, but efficacy is unaffected by broad-spectrum antibiotics.

Management of irregular bleeding

Counselling is essential and must stress that bleeding poses no risk to health and does not reflect a disease state. Interventions include short courses of a compatible combined pill or ethinyloestradiol, or the use of a short-course of tranexamic acid.

All interventions are meant to buy time and give the patient a respite from the bleeding, in the hope that amenorrhoea/oligomenorrhoea will set in, as it does, in up to 50% of long-term users.

Tips for safe practice

- Implants should only be fitted and removed by trained professionals.
- Difficult removals should only be attempted in centres with experience in and availability of ultrasound. Implanon is not radio-opaque, but can be located with either ultrasound or magnetic resonance imaging.
- Implants are safe to use in breastfeeding women with no demonstrable effect on milk volume or quality, and/or short-term infant developmental parameters.

Evidence that matters

The history of Norplant's launch in the UK and its ultimate demise is the classic "boom-and-bust" story, where hyped up contraceptives generate unrealistic expectations among users and entice professionals to offer the method without adequate counselling, resulting in a serious rebound phenomenon.

The future observed

The most interesting of the new-generation implants is nesterone, a 19-norprogesterone derivative, effective for 2 years. Nesterone is distinguished from other progestogens by not being a testosterone-derivative and being inactivated by gastric enzymes, making it the ideal progestogen contraceptive for lactating women as even the small amounts excreted in breast milk tend to be destroyed by the infant's gastric juices.

Emergency contraception

Overview

Sex is a spontaneous, often unplanned activity. Current contraceptives are not perfect and "accidents" happen. Emergency contraception (EC), be it hormone tablets or copper-bearing IUD, is a highly effective back-up when contraception fails or if sex is unprotected. Wide use of emergency hormonal contraception (EHC) in high-abortion areas can prevent as many as 60% of abortions.[187]

In countries without a licensed product, many resort to "DIY" EC using available COCs or POPs to make up the recommended effective dose.

Types of emergency contraception

The different types of EC are given in Table 25. The hormonal methods include the combined oestrogen/progestogen (Yuzpe) regimen,[188,189] which has been superseded by progestogen-only EC.[190] A further hormonal method is mifepristone, which is a highly effective alternative, currently only available in China for this indication.[191]

The combined Yuzpe method is still used in some countries. It consists of two doses of 100 µg ethinyloestradiol and 500 µg levonorgestrel each. The first dose is taken within 72 hours of intercourse and the second taken 12 hours after the first dose.[188,189] Although most hormonal EC research was based on levonorgestrel products, norethisterone-based pills in comparable doses may be as effective.

Levonorgestrel-only EC is currently the method of choice in many countries. The rise of levonorgestrel as the preferred EHC was a triumph for evidence-based medicine. Two WHO randomized clinical trials published in 1998[190] and 2002[191] triggered a shift in UK practice to levonorgestrel-only EHC, which was made available OTC in 2001 and instigated a licence change to a single stat dose regimen in 2003.

Table 25. Types of emergency contraceptives*

	Common brand names	Dosage
Progestogen-only emergency hormonal contraceptives		
Each of the two doses of progestogen-only contraceptives should contain at least 0.75 mg levonorgestrel	Levonelle-2, Norlevo Plan B, Postinor-2, Vikela (packaged and labeled for emergency contraception)	Two tablets in single dose ● Each tablet contains 0.75 mg levonorgestrel ●●
Combined emergency hormonal contraceptives		
Each of the two doses of combined oral contraceptives should contain at least 100 µg (0.10 mg) ethinyl estradiol and 500 µg (0.50 mg) levonorgestrel	E-Gen-C, Fertilan, Imediat, PC-4, Preven, Tetragynon (packaged and labeled for emergency contraception) or Eugynon 50, Neogynon, Noral, Nordoil, Ovidon, Ovral, Ovran	Two tablets per dose (2 doses) ●● Each tablet contains 0.75 µg ethinyl estradiol and either 0.25 mg or 0.50 mg levonorgestrel
	Lo/Femenal, Microgynon 30, Nordette, Ovral L, Rigevidon	Four tablets per dose x 2 ●● ●● Each tablet contains 30 µg ethinyl estradiol and either 0.15 mg or 0.30 mg levonorgestrel
Emergency Intrauterine device	Copper IUD	Insertion within 120 hours (5 days) of unprotected coitus
Antiprogestins	Mifepristone	10 mg is effective as a single dose ●

* Adapted from *Network Family Health International*, vol. 21, no. 1, 2001.

Previously, two doses of 0.75 mg each were taken 12 hours apart, with the first dose initiated within 72 hours of intercourse. The single stat dose of 1.5 mg has a 20% higher efficacy and is not associated with more side effects. 2005 should see the advent of advance provision of EHC, a deregulation likely to meet the need of at-risk groups, especially young women presenting with an STI.

Table 26. Attributes of the intrauterine device as emergency contraception
1. Failure rates extremely low
2. Effective when used up to 120 hours after intercourse
3. Effective when used up to 120 hours after the earliest calculated date of ovulation
4. The method can be used to "cover" multiple exposures because of [3] (see above)
5. Useful if hormonal methods are not suitable
6. Provides contraception for the rest of the cycle
7. Can be kept as ongoing contraception
8. Conversely can be removed with next period

A copper-bearing IUD is the most effective and versatile EC (Table 26). The contraindications that apply in general IUD use do not apply if the IUD is intended for EC only, with the one exception being the risk of infection, which is raised in emergency use. This happens especially in cases of sexual violence, intercourse for the first time, intercourse with a new partner, casual sex and intercourse with a partner returning to a relationship. In all such cases, screening for STIs, with follow-up and partner notification, go hand-in-hand with covering the IUD insertion with antibiotics.

The IUS (Mirena) is ineffective and unsuitable for EC.

Prevalence

This is difficult to estimate globally, as many couples are likely to resort to a DIY formula made up from available COCs or POPs.

In the UK, 1.5 million units of EHC were dispensed in 2002, with at least one-third of sales being OTC, 44% from a GP, and the rest from community family planning clinics.[192] 5% of women aged 16–49 years use EC once per year, 1% use it twice and 1% use it several times per year.[192] In one survey, overall, 11% of 16–49-year-olds reported using EHC, while 1% chose an IUD.

Indications

The obvious ones are unprotected intercourse and condom breakage and slippage. Special indications include covering missed pills (Figure 26).

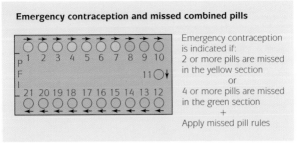

Figure 26. Emergency contraception and the missed pill.

Mechanisms of action[193]

EC methods are not abortifacient. EHC prevents or delays ovulation when taken pre-ovulation, and is likely to interfere with endometrial, ovarian and tubal mechanisms in a way that prevents/disrupts fertilization. The functionality of spermatozoa and the ovum is impeded though a number of physical and chemical changes. The emergency IUD works in a similar way at endometrial and tubal levels disrupting fertilization.

Administration and efficacy[194]

Levonelle®-2 is a licensed prescription-only-medication (POM) EC in the UK comprising two tablets of 0.75 mg levonorgestrel each, taken as a single dose any time within 72 hours from the index unprotected intercourse. Levonelle is the OTC version of EHC. The recommendation is to take the tablets as early as possible within the 72-hour window, although efficacy remains acceptable up to 120 hours (Table 27).[191]

Levonorgestrel compares well with the combined method, efficacy being less sensitive to time from exposure,[195] and having lower gastrointestinal side effects.[196]

The chances of conception vary from 20%–30% mid-cycle to nearly 0% in the immediate pre-menstrual days. Overall, a single act of intercourse carries a conception risk of 2%–4%.[191,197] No cycle day can be presumed to be 100% safe.

Table 27. Time-related efficacy of progestogen-only emergency contraception

Time since intercourse (hours)	% of expected pregnancies prevented	Successful treatment per 100 women treated
< 24	95	99.6
24–48	85	98.8
48–72	58	97.3
1–72	84	98.6
72–120	63	97.3

Efficacy can be expressed as the number of expected pregnancies prevented by EC (on average 8/10 for EHC and 9/10 for IUDs) or as percentage of successful treatment per 100 women treated (Table 27).

Attributes

EHC:

- Is extremely safe.
- Is a safety net method when other methods fail.
- Has acquired high awareness especially among young people, but awareness of the scope of the methods is still poor.

Adverse events/side effects

The only contraindications to EHC are levonorgestrel allergy, pregnancy and porphyria. All the complications inherent to an IUD fitting would apply to EC IUD.

If it is possible to fit an IUD and take measures to reduce the risk of infection, the contraindication to emergency IUDs are no different from EHC: allergy to copper and pregnancy, but not porphyria.

Table 28 shows the side effects of levonorgestrel EHC as reported in the 2002 WHO randomized clinical trial.[191]

Table 28. Frequency of side effects of levonorgestrel emergency contraception	
Side effect	% of women treated
Nausea	14
Vomiting	1
Fatigue	14
Dizziness	10
Headache	10
Mastalgia	8
Menses > 7 days early	10
Menses > 7 days late	5
Menses on time	55

Counselling points

- Assess and advise on risk of pregnancy, describe the mechanism of action and indicate the failure rates.
- Single-dose levonorgestrel is the recommended regimen for EHC.
- Highlight the attributes (and infection risk) of IUDs.
- EC is not effective if a woman is already pregnant.
- While early treatment ensures highest efficacy, EHC remains effective within the 72/120-hour window.
- Domperidone 10 mg is the antiemetic of choice if past history suggests a risk of vomiting. If vomiting occurs within 2 hours of taking the tablets, another dose or an IUD should be offered.
- Women on broad-spectrum antibiotics do not require any additional measures.
- Women on liver enzyme-inducing drugs are advised to take a stat dose of 1.5 mg levonorgestrel, followed by 0.75 mg levonorgestrel 12 hours later.
- Advise abstention or condom use until the next period.
- The failure risk is higher when intercourse, even protected, takes place post EC treatment.

- Advise on regular contraception.
- Start hormonal methods on day 1 (and up to day 5) of the next cycle.
- Immediate start of hormonal contraception makes sense as long as measures are in place to elucidate any risk of pregnancy.

Tips for safe practice

- Take a full menstrual and coital history. Exclude a pregnancy, ascertain exposure – consultation times and, if necessary, do a pregnancy test.
- EHC can be used more than once in a cycle. However, regular repeat use is associated with high failures and a 70% risk of menstrual disruption.[198]
- Multiple exposures do not contraindicate EHC. The magnitude of risk of the earliest intercourse needs to be assessed. The UK licence of Levonelle-2 allows use in multiple exposures cases.
- There is no evidence of teratogenicity when EHC fails, but no one can guarantee a normal outcome to any pregnancy.[199,200]
- There is no need to do any tests or examinations prior to prescribing EHC.
- Blood pressure and weight measurement is required if the of use hormonal contraception, such as the pill, is planned.
- Follow-up should be offered 3 weeks post-treatment, alternatively patients should be advised to return if the subsequent period is abnormal in any way or delayed over 7 days after its expected timing.
- An IUD can be removed on the first day of the next menses if the patient is anxious about side effects.
- Levonorgestrel EC is unlikely to increase the risk of ectopic pregnancy, but a recent spate of ectopic reports has raised awareness that when a pregnancy is suspected, an ectopic should be excluded.[201]

Evidence that matters

The two WHO randomized clinical trials have dispelled many of the myths and anxieties about EC. Research on mechanism of action is difficult to conduct, but is essential to enhance further the acceptance of EC by a minority who views the method as a form of abortion. Post-treatment spotting has no correlation with success or failure of EC, and does not predict the nature of subsequent menses. Treatment early in the cycle is more likely to be associated with cycle disruption.[202]

The future observed

Further deregulation of EC to ensure universal access makes sense, and does not encourage dependence on the method in place of a regular one.[203] Advance provision of one or more units of EC has the advantage that a woman can use it as soon after intercourse as she wishes, with privacy and dignity, while saving the health system scarce resources.[204] Clear written instructions/information are pre-requisites for effective use and informed choice. Access to services is essential if further EC is needed. Advance provision of EC (APEC) is covered by current UK licence. Although all women would benefit, women in contact with men with STIs may be an especially vulnerable group to target.[205]

Mifepristone is an orally active progesterone antagonist proven to be an effective EC. A minidose (10 mg) of this antiprogesterone has an efficacy comparable to levonorgestrel but with a low risk of gastrointestinal side effects. The delay of the next menses is a problem with higher doses, but not with this dose. Mifepristone, however, is not widely available.

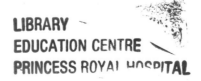

Frequently asked questions

How can I tell if I'm fertile? If so, can I use this knowledge to avoid pregnancy?

If your periods are regular, e.g. they occur every 28 days, then your fertile period is around mid-cycle, that is, day 7 to day 16 of the cycle. Since ovulation occurs 14 days before the next cycle is due, it is easier to predict the "safe" period post-ovulation for women who have a regular cycle. If your periods are irregular, you have to allow for your shortest and longest cycles. So, for cycles varying from 21 to 35 days, the potential fertile period could be between day 1 and day 23.

However, in the first half of the cycle, no day is "safe" because your partner's sperm can survive inside you for up to 7 days.

Fertility awareness methods have special instructions (*see* pp 97–103).

Do I need contraception if I'm breastfeeding?

The chance of getting pregnant is small (around 2%) if you are fully breastfeeding, if your baby is less than 6 months old, and if your periods have not restarted. However, the protective effect of breastfeeding diminishes beyond 6 months.

How effective is coitus interruptus?

Historically, withdrawal of the penis before ejaculation was the only available, "free" method of contraception. It has no serious side effects, but its effectiveness is limited, with failure rates as high as 20%. In addition, coitus interruptus may cause dissatisfaction in as many as one-third of women, as users may find it unpleasant and it may cause anxiety that withdrawal may be too late. This method is not usually promoted by family planning doctors, but it may be useful in rare situations where nothing else is available or suitable and abstention is not an option.

How effective are condoms?

Condoms can be an effective method of contraception. However, motivation and correct use are key to their success. For example, genital contact should be avoided before the condom is applied because the "pre-ejaculate" has millions of sperms. The penis should be withdrawn before it becomes flaccid to avoid spillage of semen. Be aware that sharp fingernails can tear condoms. Avoid using oil-based lubricants/treatments for some vaginal infections as these can weaken the condom.

Failure rates of only two pregnancies per 100 women years have been reported with correct and consistent use. Another benefit of condoms is the protection against STIs including HIV.

How do COCs work?

Combined oral contraceptives (COCs) contain oestrogen and a progestogen.

COCs act primarily by inhibiting ovulation. Two hormones are responsible for the development and release of an egg from the ovary: follicle-stimulating hormone (FSH) and luteinizing hormone (LH). These hormones are produced by the pituitary, a gland located at the base of the brain. FSH and LH are inhibited by COCs, so the ovary "goes to sleep".

Another mode of action of COCs is via the progestogen contained in them, which causes the cervical mucus to thicken and thus become impenetrable to sperm. It also makes the womb lining unsuitable for the sperm. So, in the very rare cases where ovulation may occur, COCs act to prevent fertilization.

How do POPs work?

Progestogen-only pills (POPs) contain progestogen alone in a much smaller amount than COCs. For this reason, they do not consistently prevent ovulation, except for the pill Cerazette. However, the high efficacy of POPs comes from their action on the cervical mucus: they greatly reduce the volume of mucus, increase its viscosity and cell content, and alter its molecular structure. These actions make the cervical mucus impenetrable to sperm and result in little or no sperm entry to the uterine cavity. Even if sperm does penetrate the mucus, sperm motility may be reduced and fertilization is unlikely.

Are there any precautions to take with POPs?

Provided that you stick to the rules relating to pill-taking, pregnancy is unlikely. However, if you forget to take your pill then there are rules that make sure you do not fall pregnant. A pill is regarded as missed if it is taken more than 3 hours late. Take the next pill as soon as possible. Additional precautions, such as condom use, are required until 48 hours after re-starting your pills. If you are on Cerazette, you have a 12-, and not 3-, hour missing window, but precautions need to be taken up to 7 days.

Antibiotics that induce liver enzymes such as rifampicin and griseofulvin make all oral pills ineffective and necessitate additional precautions. If you need to take these drugs long-term, you will require a different method of contraception.

What are long-acting hormonal contraceptives?

Unlike pills with which you need to remember to take one every day, there are contraceptives that only require you to remember to do something every week, such as the contraceptive patch, every month, such as the contraceptive vaginal ring, or every 2 to 3 months, such as the injection. Implanon, the contraceptive implant (some people call it "chip") lasts for 3 years. The hormone-releasing device ("coil") lasts for 5 years.

How effective is the levonorgestrel IUS as a method of family planning and how does it work?

This IUS is highly effective, and is associated with only 0.2 pregnancies per 100 women years. This is less than other contraceptives and comparable to female sterilization.

Mirena (the IUS) slowly releases the hormone levonorgestrel locally within the uterine cavity. Provided that it is introduced at the correct time, it becomes effective immediately. The levonorgestrel IUS offers great flexibility as fertility is immediately restored upon its removal from your uterus.

What are contraceptive implants?

These are silicon implants that slowly release a progestogen to provide contraception. Currently, Implanon is the only contraceptive implant available in the UK. In addition to thickening the cervical mucus and keeping the womb lining thin, it inhibits ovulation. Implanon is a single rod (40 mm long and 2 mm diameter) that can be easily introduced under the skin of the upper arm. Its effect lasts 3 years. It may stop periods in some users and cause infrequent spotting in others.

References

1. Oakley D. Rethinking patient counselling techniques for changing contraceptive use behavior. *Am J Obstet Gynecol* 1994;**170**: 1585–1590

2. Little P, Griffin S, Kelly J *et al*. Effect of educational leaflets and questions on knowledge of contraception in women taking the combined contraceptive pill: randomised controlled trial. *BMJ* 1998;**316**: 1948–1952

3. Jones D, Paramjit G. Breaking down language barriers. *BMJ* 1998;**316**: 1476

4. IPF International Medical Advisory Panel. IMAP statements on contraception counselling. *IPPF Med Bull* 1994;**28**: 1–3

5. Belfield T. The contraceptive decision: information and counselling. In: Kubba A, Sanfilippo J, Hampton N, eds. *Contraception and office gynecology*. London: WB Saunders, 1999.

6. Godwin K. Consumers' understanding of contraceptive efficacy. *Br J Fam Plann* 1997;**23**:45–46.

7. Vessey MP. The Jephcott lecture, 1989. An overview of the benefits of combined oral contraceptives. In: Mann RD (ed.). *Oral contraceptives and breast cancer*. New Jersey: Parthenon, 1990.

8. Kubba A, Guillebaud J, Anderson RA *et al*. Contraception. *Lancet* 2000;**356**:1913–1919

9. Schlesselman JJ. Oral contraceptives and neoplasia of the uterine corpus. *Contraception* 1991;**43**:557–559.

10. Vessey M, Villard MacKintosh L, Painter R *et al*. Epidemiology of endometriosis in women attending Family Planning Clinics. *Br Med J* 1993;**306**:182–184.

11. Levi F, Pasche C, Lucchini F, *et al*. Oral contraceptives and colorectal cancer. *Dig Liver Dis* 2003;**35**:85–87.

12. Friedman AJ, Thomas PD. Does low-dose combinationoral contraceptrive use affect uterine suze or menstrual flow in premenopausal women with leiomyomas? *Obstet Gynecol* 1995;**85**:631–635.

13. Vessey M, Metcalfe A, Wells C *et al*. Ovarian neoplasms, functional ovarian cysts and oral contraceptives. *Br Med J* 1987;**294**:1518–1520.

14. Kemmeren JM, Algra A, Grobbee DE. Third generation oral contraceptives and the risk of venous thrombosis: meta-analysis. *BMJ* 2001;**323**:131–134.

15. World Health Organization Collaborative Study of Cardiovascular Disease and Steroid Hormone Contraception. Venous thromboembolic disease and combined oral contraceptives: results of international multicentre case-control study. *Lancet* 1995;**346**:1575–1582.

16. Jick H, Jick SS, Gurewich V *et al*. Risk of idiopathic cardiovascular death and nonfatal venous thromboembolism in women using oral contraceptives with differing progestagen components. *Lancet* 1995;**346**:1589–1593.

17. Bloemenkamp KW, Rosendaal FR, Helmerhorst FM *et al*. Enhancement by factor V Leiden mutation of risk of deep-vein thrombosis associated with oral contraceptives containing a third-generation progestagen. *Lancet* 1995;**346**:1593–1596.

18. Lidegaard O, Edstrom B, Kreiner S. Oral contraceptives and venous thromboembolism. A case-control study. *Contraception* 1998;**57**:291–301.

19. Spitzer WO. The aftermath of a pill scare: regression to reassurance. *Hum Reprod Update* 1999;**5**:736–745.

20. Bloemenkamp KW, Rosendaal FR, Buller HR *et al*. Risk of venous thrombosis with use of current low-dose oral contraceptives is not explained by diagnostic suspicion and referral bias. *Arch Intern Med* 1999;**159**:65–70.

21. Vandenbroucke JP, Koster T, Briet E *et al*. Increased risk of venous thrombosis in oral contraceptive users who are carriers of factor V Leiden mutation. *Lancet* 1994;**244**:1453–1457.

22. WHO Collaborative Study of Cardiovascular Disease and Steroid Hormone Contraception. Haemorrhagic stroke, overall stroke risk and combined oral contraceptives: results of an international, multicentre, case-control study. *Lancet* 1996;**348**:505–510.

23. MacGregor A. Hormonal contraception and migraine. *J Fam Plann Reprod Health Care* 2001;**27**:49–52.

24. WHO Collaborative Study of Cardiovascular Disease and Steroid Hormone Contraception. Acute myocardial infarction and oral contraceptives: results of an international multicentre case-control study. *Lancet* 1997;**349**:1202–1209.

25. Hsing AW, Hoover RN, McLaughlin JK *et al*. Oral contraceptives and primary liver cancer among young women. *Cancer Causes Control* 1992;**3**:43–48.

26. Murray FE, Logan RF, Hannaford PC *et al*. Cigarette smoking and parity as risk factors for the development of symptomatic gall bladder diseases in women: results of the Royal College of General Practitioners' Oral Contraceptives Study. *Gut* 1994;**35**:107–111.

27. Collaborative Group on Hormonal Factors in Breast Cancer. Breast cancer and hormonal contraceptives; collaborative re-analysis of individual data on 53 297 women with breast cancer and 100 239 women without breast cancer from 54 epidemiological studies. *Lancet* 1996;**347**:1713–1727.

28. Moreno V, Bosch FX, Munoz N *et al*. Effect of oral contraceptives on the risk of cervical cancer in women with human papilloma virus infection: the IARC multicentre case-control study. *Lancet* 2002;**359**:1085–1092.

29. Smith JS, Green J, Berrington de Gonzalez A *et al*. Cervical cancer and use of hormonal contraceptives: a systematic review. *Lancet* 2003;**361**:1159–1167.

30. Meirik O. Combined oral contraceptives, human papilloma virus, and cervical cancer. *IPPF Medical Bulletin* 2002;**36**:2–3.

31. World Health Organization. Selected practice recommendations for contraceptive use. Geneva: World Health Organization, 2002.

32. Vessey M, Painter R, Yeates D. Mortality in relation to oral contraceptive use and cigarette smoking. *Lancet* 2003;**362**:185–191.

33. Elliman A. Interactions with hormonal contraception. *J Fam Plann Reprod Health Care* 2000;**26**:109–111.

34. de Souza A, Brechin S, Penney G. The members' enquiry service: frequently asked questions. *J Fam Plann Reprod Health Care* 2003;**29**:225–226.

35. Oelkers W, Foidart JM, Dombrovicz N *et al*. Effects of a new oral contraceptive containing an antimineralocorticoid progestogen, drospirenone, on the renin-aldosterone system, body weight, blood pressure, glucose tolerance, and lipid metabolism. *J Clin Endocrinol Metab* 1995;**80**:1816–1821.

36. van Vloten WA, van Haselen CW, van Zuuren EJ *et al*. The effect of 2 combined oral Contraceptives containing either drospirenone or cyproterone acetate on acne and seborrhea. *Cutis* 2002 ;**69** (Suppl. 4):2–15.

37. Foidart JM, Wuttke W, Bouw GM *et al*. A comparative investigation of contraceptive reliability, cycle control and tolerance of two monophasic oral contraceptives containing either drospirenone or desogestrel. *Eur J Contracept Reprod Health Care* 2000;**5**:124–134.

38. Huber J, Foidart JM, Wuttke W *et al*. Efficacy and tolerability of a monophasic oral contraceptive containing ethinylestradiol and drospirenone. *Eur J Contracept Reprod Health Care* 2000;**5**:25–34.

39. Borenstein J, Yu HT, Wade S *et al*. Effect of an oral contraceptive containing ethinyl estradiol and drospirenone on premenstrual symptomatology and health-related quality of life. *J Reprod Med* 2003;**48**:79–85.

40. Apter D, Borsos A, Baumgartner W *et al*. Effect of an oral contraceptive containing drospirenone and ethinylestradiol on general well-being and fluid-related symptoms. *Eur J Contracept Reprod Health Care* 2003;**8**:37–51.

41. Sillem M, Schneidereit R, Heithecker R *et al*. Use of an oral contraceptive containing drospirenone in an extended regimen. *Eur J Contracept Reprod Health Care* 2003;**8**:162–169.

42. Holt VL, Gushing-Haugen KL, Daling JR. Body weight and risk of oral contraceptive failure. *Obstet Gynecol* 2002;**99**:820–827.

43. Miller L, Hughes JP. Continuous combination oral contraceptive pills to eliminate withdrawal bleeding: a randomised trial. *Obstet Gynecol* 2003;**101**:653–661.

44. Wright KL. 'Quick Start' of pills promising. *Network* 2003;**22**:10.

45. Best K. Hormonal contraception and STIs. *Network* 2003;**22**:21.

46. Tanis BC, van den Bosch MAAJ, Kemmeren JM *et al*. Oral contraceptives and the risk of myocardial infarction. *N Engl J Med* 2001;**345**:1787–1793.

47. Lidegaard O, Kreiner S. Contraceptives and cerebral thrombosis: a five-year national case-control study. *Contraception* 2002;**65**:197–205.

48. Kemmeren JM, Tanis BC, van den Bosch MAAJ *et al*. Risk of arterial thrombosis in relation to oral contraceptives (RATIO) study. Oral contraceptives and the risk of ischemic stroke. *Stroke* 2002;**33**:1202.

49. Lidegaard O, Edstrom B, Kreiner S. Oral contraceptives and venous thromboembolism: a five-year national case-control study. *Contraception* 2002;**65**:187–196.

50. Sullivan H, Furniss H, Spona J *et al*. Effect of 21-day and 24-day oral contraceptive regimens containing gestodene (60 µg) and ethinyl estradiol (15 µg) on ovarian activity. *Fertil Steril* 1999;**72**:115–120.

51. Vessey MP, Lawless M, Yeates D, Mc Pherson K. Progestogen only contraception: findings in a large prospective study with special reference to effectiveness. *Br J Fam Plann* 1985;**10**:117.

52. World Health Organization, Task Force for Epidemiological Research on Reproductive Health. Progestogen-only contraceptives during lactation: 1. Infant growth. *Contraception* 1994;**50**:35–53.

53. Tayob Y, Adams J, Jacobs HS *et al*. Ultrasound demonstration of increased frequency of functional ovarian cysts in women using progestogen only oral contraception. *Br J Obstet Gynecol* 1985;**92**:1003.

54. Franks AL, Beral V, Cates W Jr *et al*. Contraception and ectopic pregnancy risk. *Am J Obstet Gynecol* 1990;**163**:1120.

55. Vessey MP, Mears E, Andolsek L *et al*. Randomised double blind trial of four oral progestogen-only contraceptives. *Lancet* 1972;**1**:915–922.

56. de Souza A, Brechin S, Penney G. The members' enquiry service: frequently asked questions. *J Fam Plann Reprod Health Care* 2003;**29**:160–161.

57. Faculty of family planning and reproductive health care. New product review: desogestrel-only pill (cerazette), 2003.

58. Rice CF, Killick SR, Dieben TOM *et al*. A comparison of the inhibition of ovulation achieved by desogestrel 75 micrograms and levonorgestrel 30 micrograms daily. *Human reproduction* 1999;**14**:982–985.

59. Rice C, Killick S, Hickling D *et al*. Ovarian activity and vaginal bleeding patterns with a desogestrel – only preparation at three different doses. *Hum Reprod* 1996;**11**:737–740.

60. Collaborative Study Group on the desogestrel-containing progestogen-only pill: a double-blind study comparing the contraceptive efficacy, acceptability and safety of two progestogen-only pills containing desogestrel 75 µg/day or levonorgestrel 30 µg/day. *Eur J Contracept Reprod Health Care* 1998;**3**:169–178.

61. Bjarnadottir RI, Gottfredsdottir H, Sigurdardotter K *et al*. Comparative study of the effects of a progestogen-only pill containing desogestreland an intrauterine device in lactating women. *Br J Obstet Gynaecol* 2001;**108**:1174–1180.

62. Benagiano G, Primiero FM. Long-acting contraceptives. Present status. *Drugs* 1983;**25**:570–609.

63. De Ceular K, Gruber C, Hayes R *et al*. Medroxy-progesterone acetate and homozygous sickle cell disease. *Lancet* 1982;**2**:229.

64. Mattson R, Cramer J, Caldwell B *et al*. Treatment of seizures with medroxy-progesterone acetate: preliminary report. *Neurology* 1984;**34**:1255.

65. World Health Organization. Collaborative Study of Neoplasia and Steroid Contraceptives. Depot medroxyprogesterone acetate (DMPA) and risk of endometrial cancer. *Int J Cancer* 1991;**49**:186–190.

66. Gbolade BA. Depo-provera and bone density. *J Fam Plann Reprod Health Care* 2002;**28**:7–11.

67. Petitti DB, Piaggio J, Mehta S *et al.*, for the WHO study of hormonal contraception and bone health. Steroid hormone contraception and bone mineral density: a cross-sectional study in an international population. *Obstet Gynecol* 2000;**97**:736–744.

68. Sorensen MB, Collins P, Ong P *et al.* Long-term use of contraceptive depot medroxyprogesterone acetate in young women impairs arterial endothelial function assessed by cardiovascular magnetic resonance. *Circulation* 2002;**106**:1646–1651.

69. Clark MK, Sowers M, Levy BT *et al.* Magnitude and variability of sequential estradiol and progesterone concentrations in women using depot medroxyprogesterone acetate for contraception. *Fertil Steril* 2001;**75**:871–877.

70. Skegg DCG, Noonan EA, Paul C *et al.* Depot medroxyprogesterone acetate and breast cancer: a pooled analysis of the World Health Organization and New Zealand studies. *JAMA* 1995;**273**:799–804.

71. Shapiro S, Rosenberg L, Hoffman M *et al.* Risk of breast cancer in relation to the use of injectable progestogen contraceptives and combined estrogen/progestogen contraceptives. *Am J Epidemiol* 2000;**151**:396–403.

72. Baeten JM, Nyange P, Richardson BA *et al.* Hormonal contraception and risk of sexually transmitted disease acquisition: results from a prospective study. *Am J Obstet Gynecol* 2001;**185**:380–385.

73. Scholes D, La Croix AZ, Ichikkawa LE *et al.* The association between depot medroxyprogesterone contraception and bone mineral density in adolescent women. *Contraception* 2004;**69**:99–104.

74. Cundy T, Cornish J, Roberts H *et al.* Menopausal bone loss in long-term users of depot medroxyprogesterone acetate contraception. *Am J Obstet Gynecol* 2002;**186**:978–983.

75. Cromer BA. Bone mineral density in adolescent and young adult women on injectable or oral contraception. Current opinion in obstetrics and gynaecology 2003;**15**:353–357.

76. UN/WHO Task Force on Long Acting Systemic Agents for Fertility Regulation. Comparative study of the effects of two once-a-month injectable contraceptives (cyclofem and mesigyna) and one oral contraceptive (ortho-novum 1/35) on coagulation and fibrinolysis. *Contraception* 2003;**68**:159–176.

77. Muller N. Self-injection with Cyclofem. *Int Planned Parenthood Fed Med Bull* 1998;**32**:1–3.

78. Family Health International. Barrier methods. *Network* 1996;**16** (3).

79. Weller S, Davis K. Condom effectiveness in reducing heterosexual HIV transmission. *Cochrane Database Syst Rev* 2002;**1**:CD003255.

80. Trussell J, Hatcher RA, Cates W *et al*. Contraceptive failure in the United States: an update. *Stud Fam Plann* 1990;**21**:51–54.

81. Bounds W, Molloy S, Guillebaud J. Pilot study of short-term acceptability and breakage and slippage rates for the loose-fitting polyurethane male condom eZ.on bi-directional: a randomized cross-over trial. *Eur J Contracept Reprod Health Care* 2002;**7**:71–78.

82. Gallo MF, Grimes DA, Schulz KF. Nonlatex vs latex male condoms for contraception: a systematic review of randomized controlled trials. *Contraception* 2003;**68**:319–326.

83. Coker AL, Hulka BS, McCann MF *et al*. Barrier methods of contraception and cervical intraepithelial neoplasia. *Contraception* 1992;**45**:1–10.

84. Hogewoning CJA, Bleeker MCG, Van der Brule AJC *et al*. Condom use promotes regression of cervical intraepithelial neoplasia and clearance of human papilloma virus: a randomized clinical trial. *Int J Cancer* 2003;**107**:811–816.

85. Trussell J, Warner DL, Hatcher RA. Condom slippage and breakage rates. *Fam Plann Perspect* 1992;**25**:20–23.

86. Steiner M, Piedrahita C, Glover L *et al*. Can condom users likely to experience condom failure be identified? *Fam Plann Perspect* 1993;**25**:22–223.

87. Richters J, Gerofi J, Donovan B. Why do condoms break or slip off in use? An exploratory study. *Int J STD AIDS* 1995;**6**:11–18.

88. Sparrow MJ, Lavil K. Breakage and slippage of condoms in family planning clients. *Contraception* 1994;**50**:117–129.

89. Gabbay M, Gibbs A. Does additional lubrication reduce condom failure? *Contraception* 1996;**53**:155–158.

90. Webb A. The female condom – a reappraisal three years on (editorial). *Br J Fam Plann* 1996;**21**:27.

91. Trussell J, Sturgen K, Strickler J *et al*. Comparartive contraceptive efficacy of the female condom and other barrier methods. *Fam Plann Perspect* 1994;**26**:66–72.

92. Roddy RE, Zekeng L, Ryan KA *et al*. Effect of nonoxynol- 9 Gel on urogenital gonorrhea and chlamydia infections. *JAMA* 20002;**287**:1117–1122.

93. Van Damme L, Ramjee G, Alary M *et al*. Effectiveness of Col-1492, a nonoxynol-9 vaginal Gel, on HIV-1 transmission in female sex workers: a randomized controlled trial. *Lancet* 2002;**360**:971–977.

94. Centers for Disease Control and Prevention. Sexually transmitted diseases treatment guidelines. *Morbidity and Mortality Weekly Report* 2002;**51**(RR-6):1–80.

95. Trussell J, Stricker J, Vaughan B. Contraceptive efficacy of the diaphragm, the sponge and the cervical cap. *Fam Plann Perspect* 1993;**25**:100–105.

96. Fihn SD, Latham RH, Roberts P *et al*. Association between diaphragm use and urinary tract infection. *JAMA* 1985;**254**:240–245.

97. Richwald GA, Greenland S, Gerber M *et al*. Effectiveness of the cavity-rim cervical cap: results of a large clinical study. *Obstet Gynecol* 1989;**74**:143–148.

98. Mauck C, Glover LH, Miller E. Lea's shield®: a study of the safety and efficacy of a new vaginal barrier contraceptive used with and without spermicide. *Contraception* 1996;**53**:329–335.

99. Shihati AA, Gollub E. Acceptability of a new intravaginal barrier contraceptive device (FemCap). *Contraception* 1992;**46**:511–519.

100. Psychoyos A. Protectaid, a new vaginal contraceptive sponge with anti-STD properties. In: *Barrier contraceptive*: current status and future prospects. New York: Wiley-Liss, Inc., 1994.

101. Creatsas G, Elsheikh A, Colin P. Safety and tolerability of the new contraceptive sponge Protectaid. *Eur J Contracept Reprod Health Care* 2002;**7**:91–95.

102. WHO Scientific Group. Mechanisms of action, safety and efficacy of intrauterine devices. Tech Rep Ser 753. Geneva: World Health Organization, 1987.

103. United Nations Development Programme/United Nations Population Fund/WHO/World Bank. Long-term reversible contraception: twelve years of experience with the Tcu380A and T220C. *Contraception* 1997;**56**:341–352.

104. Grimes D, Shulz K, Van Vlict H *et al*. Immediate post-partum insertion of intrauterine devices. A Cochrane Review. *Hum Reprod* 2002;**17**:549–453.

105. Grimes D, Schulz K, Stanwood N. Immediate postabortal insertion of intrauterine devices (Cochrane Review). *The Cochrane Library*. Issue 4, 2003. Chichester: John Wiley & Sons Ltd.

106. Faculty of family planning and reproductive health care. Clinical Effectiveness Unit. The copper intrauterine device as a long-term contraception. *J Fam Plann Reprod Health Care* 2004;**30**:29–42.

107. Hubacher D, Grimes DA. Noncontraceptive health benefits of intrauterine devices: a systemic review. *Obstet Gynecol Surv* 2002;**57**:120–128.

108. Fraley TNM, Rosenberg MJ, Rose PJ *et al*. Intrauterine devices and pelvic inflammatory disease: an international perspective. *Lancet* 1992;**339**:785–788.

109. Grimes D. Intrauterine device and upper-genital-tract infection. *Lancet* 2000;**356**:1013–1019.

110. Sivin I. Dose and age dependent ectopic pregnancy risks with intrauterine contraception. Obstet Gynecol 1991;78:291–298.

111. Clinical and Scientific Committee Faculty of Family Planning & Reproductive Healthcare of the RCOG. Recommendations for clinical practice: Actinomyces like organisms and intrauterine contraceptives. *Br J Fam Plann* 1998;**23**:137–138.

112. Walsh T, Grimes D, Frezieres R *et al*. Randomised controlled trial of prophylactic antibiotics before insertion of intrauterine devices. *Lancet* 1998;**351**:1005–1008.

113. Grimes DA. Intrauterine devices and infertility: sifting through the evidence. *Lancet* 2001;**358**:6–7.

114. Anon. Frameless intra-uterine contraceptive device (GyneFix). *Drug Ther Bull* 2002;**40**:21–22.

115. Masters T, Everret S, May M *et al*. Outcomes at 1 year for the first 200 patients fitted with the GyneFix at the Margaret Pyke Centre. *Eur J Contracept Reprod Health Care* 2002;**7**:65–70.

116. Nilsson CG, Lahteenmaki P, Luukkainen T. Levonorgestrel plasma concentrations and hormone profiles after insertion and after one year of treatment with a levonorgestrel-IUD. *Contraception* 1980;**21**:225–233.

117. Nilsson CG, Pertti L, Lahteenmaki A *et al*. Ovarian function in amenorrhoeic and menstruating users of a levonorgestrel-releasing device. *Fertil Steril* 1984;**41**:52–55.

118. Rowlands S, Hampton N. Intrauterine contraception. In: *Contraception and Office Gynecology*. Kubba A, Sanfilippo J, Hampton N (eds). London: WB Saunders, 1999.

119. Anon. A plethora of IUDs: but how safe, how effective? *Prog Reprod Health Res* 2002;**60**:3.

120. Bounds W, Guillebaud J. Observational series on women using the contraceptive Mirena concurrently with the anti-epileptic and other enzyme-inducing drugs. *J Fam Plann Reprod Health Care* 2002;**28**:78–80.

121. Backman T, Huhtala S, Luoto R *et al*. Advance information improves user satisfaction with the levonorgestrel intrauterine system. *Obstet Gynaecol* 2002;**99**:608–613.

122. Anderson K, Odlind V, Rybo G. Levonorgestrel-releasing and copper-releasing (Nova T) IUDs during five years of use: a randomised comparative trial. *Contraception* 1994;**49**:56–72.

123. Silvin I, Stern J. Health during prolonged use of levonorgestrel 20 mg/d and the copper Tcu 380Ag intrauterine contraceptive devices: a multicenter study. *Fertil Steril* 1994;**61**:70–77.

124. Anderson JK, Rybo G. Levonorgestrel-releasing intrauterine device in the treatment of menorrhagia. *Br J Obstet Gynaecol* 1990;**97**:690–694.

125. Barrington JW, Bowen-Simpkins P. The levonorgestrel intrauterine system in the management of menorrhagia. *Br J Obstet Gynaecol* 1997;**104**:614–616.

126. Hurskainen R, Teperi J, Rissanen P *et al*. Quality of life and cost-effectiveness of levonorgestrel-releasing intrauterine system versus hysterectomy for treatment of menorrhagia: a randomised trial. *Lancet* 2001;**357**:273–277.

127. Barrington JW, Arunkalaivanan AS, Abdel-Fattah ME. Comparison between the levonorgestrel intrauterine system and thermal balloon ablation in the treatment of menorrhagia. *Eur J Obstet Gynecol Repro Biol* 2003;**108**:72–74.

128. Luukkainen T. Issues to debate on the Women's Health Initiative Study. *Hum Reprod* 2003;**18**:1559–1561.

129. Varila E, Wahlstrom T, Rauramo I. A 5-year follow-up study on the use of levonorgestrel intrauterine system in women receiving hormone replacement therapy. *Fertil Steril* 2001;**76**:969–973.

130. Starczewski A, Iwanicki M. [Intrauterine therapy with levonorgestrel releasing IUD of women with hypermenorrhea secondary to uterine fibroids]. *Ginekol Pol* 2000;**71**:1221–1225.

131. Gardner FJE, Konje JC, Abrams KR *et al*. Endometrial protection for tamoxifen-stimulated changes by a levonorgestrel-releasing intrauterine system: a randomised controlled trial. *Lancet* 200;**356**:1711–1717.

132. Griogorieva V, Chen-Mok M, Tarasova M *et al*. Use of a levonorgestrel-releasing intrauterine system to treat bleeding related to uterine leiomyomas. *Fertil Steril* 2003;**79**:1194–1198.

133. Fedele L, Bianchini S, Raffaelli R *et al*. Treatment of adenomyosis-associated menorrhagia with a levonorgestrel-releasing intrauterine device. *Fertil Steril* 1997;**68**:426–429.

134. Robinson GE, Bounds W, Kubba AA *et al*. Functional ovarian cysts associated with the levonorgestrel releasing intrauterine device. *Br J Fam Plann* 1989;**14**:132.

135. Zalel Y, Shulman A, Lidor A *et al*. The local progestational effect of the levonorgestrel-releasing intrauterine system: a sonographic and Doppler flow study. *Hum Reprod* 2002;**17**:2878–2880.

136. Skee D, Abrams LS, Natarajan T *et al*. Pharmacokinetics of a contraceptive patch at 4 application sites. *Clin Pharmacol Ther* 2000;**67**:159. Abstract PIII-71.

137. Smallwood G, Meador ML, Lenihan JP *et al*. Efficacy and safety of a transdermal contraceptive system. *Obstet Gynecol* 2001:**98**:799–805.

138. Hedon B, Helmerhost FM, Cronje HS *et al*. Comparison of efficacy, cycle control, compliance, and safety in users of a contraceptive patch vs an oral contraceptive. *Int J Gynaecol Obstet* 2000;**70** (Suppl. 1):78. Abstract FC 2.30.06.

139. Audet M-C, Moreau M, Koltun WD *et al*. Evaluation of contraceptive efficacy and cycle control of a transdermal contraceptive patch vs. an oral contraceptive. *JAMA* 2001;**285**:2347–2354.

140. Fu H, Darrroch JE, Haas T *et al*. Contraceptive failure rates, new estimates from the 1995 national survey of family growth. *Fam Plann Perspect* 1999;**31**:56–63.

141. Abrams LS. Phramacokinetics of norelgestromine and ethinylestradiol delivered by a contraceptive patch under conditions of heat, humidity and exercise. *J Clin Pharmacol* 2001;**41**:1301–1309.

142. Archer DF, Cullins V, Creasy GW *et al*. The impact of improved compliance with a weekly contraceptive transdermal system (ortho evra) on contraceptive efficacy. *Contraception* 2004;**69**:189–195.

143. Abrams LS, Skee D, Natarajan J *et al*. Tetracycline HCL does not affect the pharmacokinetics of a contraceptive patch. *Int J Gynecol Obstet* 2000;**70** (Suppl. 1):57–58.

144. Oger E, Alhenc-Gilas M, Lacut K *et al*. Differential effect of oral and transdermal estrogen/progesterone regimens on sensitivity to activated protein C among postmenopausal women. *Arterioscler Thromb Vac Biol* 2003:**23**:1671–1676.

145. Gallo MF, Grimes DA,Shulz KF. Skin patch and vaginal ring versus combined oral contraceptives for contraception (Cochrane Review). *The Cochrane Library*. Issue 3, 2003. Chichester: John Wiley & Sons Ltd.

146. Diaz S. Contraceptive vaginal rings. *Int Planned Parenthood Fed Med Bull* 1999;**33**:3–4.

147. Dieben TO, Roumen FJ, Apter D. Efficacy, cycle control and user acceptability of a novel combined contraceptive vaginal ring. *Obtset Gynecol* 2002;**100**:585–593.

148. Roumen FJ, Apter D, Mulders TM *et al*. Efficacy, tolerability and acceptability of a novel contraceptive vaginal ring releasing etonorgestrel and ethinyl oestradiol. *Hum Reprod* 2001;**16**:469–475.

149. Novak A, de la Loge C, Abetz L *et al*. The combined contraceptive vaginal ring, NuvaRing: an international study of user acceptability. *Contraception* 2003;**67**:187–194.

150. Bjarnadottir RI, Tuppurainen M, Killick SR. Comparison of cycle control with a combined contraceptive vaginal ring and oral levonorgestrel/ethinyl estradiol. *Am J Obstet Gynecol* 2002;**186**:389–395.

151. Timmer CJ, Mulders TMT. Pharmacokinetics of etonogestrel and ethinyloestradiolreleased from a combined contraceptive vaginal ring. *Clin Pharmacokinet* 2000;**39**:233–242.

152. Royal College of Obstetricians and Gynaecologists. Male and female sterilisation– evidence-based clinical guidelines no. 4. London: RCOG, 2004.

153. Rowlands S, Hannaford P. The incidence of sterilisation in the UK. *Br J Obstet Gynaecol* 2003;**110**:819–824.

154. Wilcox LS, Chu SY, Peterson HB. Characteristics of women who considered or obtained tubal reanastomosis: results from a prospective study of tubal sterilization. *Obstet Gynecol* 1990;**75**:661–665.

155. Miracle-McMahill HL, Calle EE, Kosinski AS *et al.* Tubal ligation and fatal ovarian cancer in a large prospective cohort study. *Am J Epidemiol* 1997;**145**:349–357.

156. Norad SA, Sun P,Ghodirian P *et al.* Tubal ligation and risk of ovarian cancer in carriers of BRCA1 or BRCA2 mutation: a case-control study. *Lancet* 2001;**357**:1467–1470.

157. Wilcoz LS, Chu SY, Eaker ED *et al.* Risk factors for regret after tubal sterilization: 5 years of follow-up in prospective study. *Fertil Steril* 1991;**55**:927–933.

158. Thomson JA, Lincoln PJ, Mortimer P. Paternity by a seemingly infertile vasectomised man. *Br Med J* 1993;**307**:299–300.

159. Giovannucci E, Tosteson TD, Speizer FE *et al.* A long-term study of mortality in men who have undergone vasectomy. *N Engl J Med* 1992;**326**:1392–1398.

160. Schwingl PJ, Guess HA. Vasectomy and cancer: an update. *Gynaecol Forum* 1996;**1**:24–28.

161. Cox B, Sneyd MJ, Paul C *et al.* Vasectomy and risk of prostate cancer. *JAMA* 2002;**287**:3110–3115.

162. Chen-Mok M,Bbangdiwala SI, Dominik R *et al.* Termination of a randomised controlled trial of two vasectomy techniques. *Control Clin Trials* 2003;**24**:78–84.

163. Li S, Goldstein M, Zhu J *et al.* The no-scalpel vasectomy. *J Urol* 1991;**145**:341–344.

164. Engender Health. No-scalpel vasectomy: an illustrated guide for surgeons, 3rd ed. New York: Engender Health, 2003.

165. Cooper JM, Carignan CS, Cher D *et al.* Microinsert nonincisional hysteroscopic sterilization. *Obstet Gynecol* 2003;**102**:54–67.

166. NICE. Hysteroscopic sterilisation by tubal cannulation and placement of intrafallopian implants, 2004. www.nice.org.uk.

167. Mackenzie IZ, Turner E. Sterilisation needs in the 1990s: the case for quinacrine nonsurgical female sterilisation. *Am J Obstet Gynecol* 1981;**88**:655–662.

168. El Kady AA, Nagib HS, Kessel E. Efficacy and safety of repreated transcervical quinacrine pellet insertions for female sterilization. *Fertil Steril* 1993;**59**:301–304.

169. Peterson HB, Zhisen X, Hughes JM *et al*. The risk of pregnancy after tubal sterilisation: findings from the US Collaborative Review of Sterilisation. *Am J Obstet Gynecol* 1996;**174**:1161–1170.

170. Wilcox AJ, Weinberg CR, Baird DD. Timing of sexual intercourse in relation to ovulation. *N Engl J Med* 1995;**333**: 1517-21.

171. World Health Organization. A prospective multicenter trial of the ovulation method of natural family planning 111. Characteristics of the menstrual cycle and of the fertile phase. *Fertil Steril* 1983;**40**:773–777.

172. Kerin JF, Edmonds DK, Warnes GM *et al*. Morphological and functional relations of graafian follicle growth to ovulation in women using ultrasonic, laparoscopic and biochemical measurements. *Br J Ostet Gynaecol* 1981;**88**:81–90.

173. Ryder B, Campbell H. Natural family planning in the 1980s. *Lancet* 1995;**345**:233–234.

174. Marshall J. A field-trial of the basal body temperature method of regulating births. *Lancet* 1968;**2**:8–10.

175. Keefe EF. Self-observation of the cervix to distinguish days of possible fertility. *Bull. Sloane Hosp. Women* 1962;**8**:129–136.

176. Billings JJ. The ovulation method. Melbourne: Advocate Press, 1964.

177. Bonnar J, Flynn AM, Freundl G *et al*. Personal hormone monitoring for contraception. *Br J Fam Plan*. 1999;**24**:128–134.

178. Perez A, Labbok M, Queenan J. Clinical study of the lactational amenorrhea method in family planning. *Lancet* 1992;**339**:968–970.

179. Labbok M, Perez A, Valdes V *et al*. The lactational amenorrhea method (LAM): a postpartum introductory family planning method with policy and program implications. *Adv Contracept* 1994;**10**:93–109.

180. Cooney K, Hoser H, Labbok M. Assessment of the nine month LAM method experience in Rwanda (Presentation and Abstract). American Public Health Annual Meeting, October 1993.

181. Darney P, Speroff L. Implant comtraception. In: Darney P, Speroff L. (eds) *A clinical guide for contraception*, 2nd ed. Baltimore: Williams and Wilkins, 1996.

182. Sivin I, Viegas O, Compodonico I *et al*. Clinical performance of a new two-rod levonorgestrel contraceptive implant: a three-year randomized study with Norplant implants as controls. *Contraception* 1997;**55**:73–80.

183. Edwards J, Moore A. Implanon: a review of clinical studies. *Br J Fam Plann* 1999;**24**:S1–16.

184. Croxatto HB. Mechanisms that explain the contraceptive action of progestin implants for women. *Contraception* 2002;**65**:21–28.

185. Glassier A. Implantable contraceptives for women: effectiveness, discontinuation rates, return of fertility, and outcome of pregnancies. *Contraception* 2002;**65**:29–38.

186. Meirik O, Fraser I, d'Arcangues C for the WHO Consultation on Implantable Contraceptives for Women. Implantable contraceptives for women. *Hum Reprod Update* 2003;**9**:1–11.

187. IPPF International Medical Advisory Panel. Statement on emergency contraception. *IPPF Medical Bulletin* 2004;**38**:1–3.

188. Yuzpe AA, Lance WJ. Ethinylestradiol and DL-norgestrel as a post-coitel contraceptive. *Fertil Steril* 1977;**28**:932–936.

189. Yuzpe AA, Percival Smith R, Rademaker AW. A multi-center investigation employing ethinylestradiol combined with DL-norgestrel as a post-coitel contraceptive agent. *Fertil Steril* 1982;**37**:508–513.

190. Task Force on Postovulatory Methods of Fertility Regulation Randomised, controlled trial of levonorgestrel versus the Yuzpe regimen of combined oral contraceptives for emergency contraception. *Lancet* 1998;**352**:428–433.

191. Von Hertzen H, Piaggia G, Ding J *et al.* Low dose mifepristone and two regimens of levonorgestrel for emergency contraception: a WHO multicentre randomised trial. *Lancet* 2002;**360**:1803–1810.

192. Office for National Statistics. Contraception and sexual health 2002. London: Office for National Statistics, 2003.

193. Croxatto HB. Emergency contraception pills:how do they work? *IPPF Medical Bulletin* 2002;**36**:1–2.

194. Anon. Faculty of Family Planning and Reproductive Health Care. Royal College of Obstetricians and Gynaecologists. Guidance April 2000. Emergency contraception: recommendations for clinical practice. *Br J Fam Plann* 2000;**26**:93–96.

195. Piaggio G, von Hertzen H, Grimes DA *et al.* on behalf of the Task Force on Postovulatory Methods of Fertility Regulation. Timing of emergency contraception with levonorgestrel or the Yuzpe regimen. *Lancet* 1999;**353**:731.

196. Task Force on Postovulatory Methods of Fertility Regulation Randomised, controlled trial of levonorgestrel versus the Yuzpe regimen of combined oral contraceptives for emergency contraception. *Lancet* 1998;**352**:428–433.

197. Wilcox AJ, Dunson DB, Weinberg CR *et al.* Likelihood of conception with a single act of intercourse: providing benchmark rates for assessment of post-coital contraceptives. *Contraception* 2002;**63**:211–215.

198. UNDP/UNFPA/WHO/World Bank Special Programme of Research Development and Research Training in Human Reproduction, Task Force on Post-Ovulatory Methods of Fertility Regulation. Efficacy and side effects of immediate postcoital levonorgestrel used repeatedly for contraception. *Contraception* 2000;**61**:303–308.

199. Dixon GW, Schlesselmn JJ, Ory HW *et al*. Ethinylestradiol and conjugated estrogens on post-coital contraceptives. *JAMA* 1980;**244**:1336–1339.

200. Raman-Wilms L, Tseng AL, Wighard TS *et al*. Fetal genital effects of first-trimester sex hormone exposure;a metaanalysis. *Obstet Gynecol* 1995;**85**:141–149.

201. Black K, Kubba A. Is there a link between ectopic pregnancy and progestogen-only emergency contraception. *Trends in Urology Gynaecology and Sexual Health* 2003;**8**:5–6.

202. Webb A, Shochet T, Bigrigg A *et al*. Effect of hormonal emergency contraception on bleeding patterns. *Contraception* 2004;**69**:133–135.

203. Jackson RA, Schwartz B, Freedman L *et al*. Advance supply of emergency contraception: effect on use and usual contraception – a randomised trial. *Obstet Gynecol* 2004;**102**:8–16.

204. Glasier A, Baird D. The effects of self-administering emergency contraception. *N Engl J Med* 1998;**339**:1–4.

205. Golden MR, Whittington WL, Handsfield HH *et al*. Failure of family planning referral and high interest in advanced provision emergency contraception among women contacted for STD partner notification. *Contraception* 2004;**69**:241–246.

Appendix 1 – WHO medical eligibility for contraceptive use

WHO Medical Eligibility Criteria – a tool to balance the risks and benefits of any contraceptive within a wide range of conditions

WHO eligibility criteria*†

Category 1: A condition for which there is no restriction for the use of the contraceptive method

Category 2: A condition where the advantages of the method generally outweigh the risks

Category 3: A condition where the theoretical or proven risks usually outweigh the advantages of using the method

Category 4: A condition that represents an unacceptable health risk if the contraceptive method is used

*World Health Organization. *Improving access to quality care in family planning*. Geneva: World Health Organization, 1996, 2000.
†Some Category 4 or 3 contra-indications to use of combined oral contraceptives (COCs) by women with specific uncommon conditions and diseases (e.g. sickle cell disease, porphyria, disorders hepatic secretion, otosclerosis) are listed in the Summaries of Product Characteristics and the British National Formulary. However, for many such uncommon conditions there is no direct research evidence of the effect of COCs.

Condition	Combined oral contraceptives	Combined injectable contraceptives	Progestogen-only pills	Depot-medroxy-progesterone acetate Norethisterone enanthate	Norplant and Norplant II implants	Copper intrauterine devices	Levonorgestrel intrauterine devices
Personal characteristics and reproductive history							
Pregnancy	NA	NA	NA	NA	NA	4	4
Age	Menarche to < 40 = 1 ≥ 40 = 2	Menarche to < 40 = 1 ≥ 40 = 2	Menarche to < 18 = 1 18–45 = 1 > 45 = 1	Menarche to < 18 = 2 18–45 = 1 > 45 = 2	Menarche to < 18 = 1 18–45 = 1 > 45 = 1	< 20 = 2 ≥ 20 = 1	< 20 = 2 ≥ 20 = 1

Condition	Combined oral contraceptives	Combined injectable contraceptives	Progestogen-only pills	Depot-medroxy-progesterone acetate Norethisterone enanthate	Norplant and Norplant II implants	Copper intrauterine devices	Levonorgestrel intrauterine devices
Personal characteristics and reproductive history							
Parity							
a) Nulliparous	1	1	1	1	1	2	2
b) Parous	1	1	1	1	1	1	1
Breastfeeding							
a) < 6 weeks postpartum	4	4	3	3	3		
b) 6 weeks to < 6 months (primarily breastfeeding)	3	3	1	1	1		
c) ≥ 6 months postpartum	2	2	1	1	1		
Postpartum (in non-breastfeeding women)							
a) < 21 days	3	3	1	1	1		
b) ≥ 21 days	1	1	1	1	1		

Condition	Combined oral contraceptives	Combined injectable contraceptives	Progestogen-only pills	Depot-medroxy-progesterone acetate Norethisterone enanthate	Norplant and Norplant II implants	Copper intrauterine devices	Levonorgestrel intrauterine devices
Personal characteristics and reproductive history							
Postpartum (breastfeeding or non-breastfeeding) including post-caesarean section							
a) < 48 hours						2	3
b) 48 hours to < 4 weeks						3	3
c) ≥ 4 weeks						1	1[1]
d) Puerperal sepsis						4	4
Post-abortion							
a) First trimester	1	1	1	1	1	1	1
b) Second trimester	1	1	1	1	1	2	2
c) Immediate post-septic abortion	1	1	1	1	1	4	4
Past ectopic pregnancy	1	1	2	1	1	1	1

[1] If the woman is breastfeeding, levonorgestrel intrauterine device becomes category 3 until 6 weeks postpartum

Condition	Combined oral contraceptives	Combined injectable contraceptives	Progestogen-only pills	Depot-medroxyprogesterone acetate Norethisterone enanthate	Norplant and Norplant II implants	Copper intrauterine devices	Levonorgestrel intrauterine devices
Personal characteristics and reproductive history							
History of pelvic surgery (see also *Postpartum* section) (including *Caesarean* section)	1	1	1	1	1	1	1
Smoking							
a) Age < 35	2	2					
b) Age ≥ 35							
i) < 15 cigarettes/day	3	2	1	1	1	1	1
ii) ≥ 15 cigarettes/day	4	3	1	1	1	1	1
Obesity ≥ 30 kg/m² body mass index (BMI)	2	2	1	1	1	1	1

Condition	Combined oral contraceptives	Combined injectable contraceptives	Progestogen-only pills	Depot-medroxy-progesterone acetate Norethisterone enanthate	Norplant and Norplant II implants	Copper intrauterine devices	Levonorgestrel intrauterine devices
Personal characteristics and reproductive history							
Anatomical abnormalities a) That distort the uterine cavity b) That do not distort the uterine cavity						4 2	4 2
Blood pressure measurement unavailable	NA	NA	NA	NA	NA	NA	NA
Cardiovascular disease							
Multiple risk factors for arterial cardiovascular disease (e.g. older age, smoking, diabetes and hypertension)	3/4	3/4	2	3	2	1	2

Condition	Combined oral contraceptives	Combined injectable contraceptives	Progestogen-only pills	Depot-medroxy-progesterone acetate Norethisterone enanthate	Norplant and Norplant II implants	Copper intrauterine devices	Levonorgestrel intrauterine devices
Cardiovascular disease							
Hypertension							
a) History of hypertension where blood pressure CANNOT be evaluated (including hypertension during pregnancy)	3	3	2	2	2	1	2
b) Adequately controlled hypertension, where blood pressure CAN be evaluated	3	3	1	2	1	1	1
c) Elevated blood pressure (properly taken measurements)							
i) systolic 140–159 or diastolic 90–99	3	3	1	2	1	1	1
ii) systolic ≥ 160 or diastolic ≥ 100	4	4	2	3	2	1	2
d) Vascular disease	4	4	2	3	2	1	2

Condition	Combined oral contraceptives	Combined injectable contraceptives	Progestogen-only pills	Depot-medroxy-progesterone acetate Norethisterone enanthate	Norplant and Norplant II implants	Copper intrauterine devices	Levonorgestrel intrauterine devices
Cardiovascular disease							
History of high blood pressure during pregnancy (where current blood pressure is measurable and normal)	2	2	1	1	1	1	1
Deep vein thrombosis (DVT)/Pulmonary embolism (PE)							
a) History of DVT/PE	4	4	2	2	2	1	2
b) Current DVT/PE	4	4	3	3	3	1	3
c) Family history (first-degree relatives)	2	2	1	1	1	1	1
d) Major surgery							
i) with prolonged immobilization	4	4	2	2	2	1	2
ii) without prolonged immobilization	2	2	1	1	1	1	1
e) Minor surgery without immobilization	1	1	1	1	1	1	1

Condition	Combined oral contraceptives	Combined injectable contraceptives	Progestogen-only pills	Depot-medroxy-progesterone acetate Norethisterone enanthate	Norplant and Norplant II implants	Copper intrauterine devices	Levonorgestrel intrauterine devices
Cardiovascular disease							
Superficial venous thrombosis							
a) Varicose veins	1	1	1	1	1	1	1
b) Superficial thrombophlebitis	2	2	1	1	1	1	1
Current and history of ischaemic heart disease	4	4	I 2 / C 3	3	I 2 / C 3	1	I 2 / C 3
Stroke (history of cerebro-vascular accident)	4	4	I 2 / C 3	3	I 2 / C 3	1	2
Known hyperlipidaemias (screening is NOT necessary for safe use of contraceptive)	2/3[2]	2/3[2]	2	2	2	1	2

I = initiation; **C** = continuation   [2] Depending on severity of condition

Condition	Combined oral contraceptives		Combined injectable contraceptives		Progestogen-only pills		Depot-medroxy-progesterone acetate Norethisterone enanthate		Norplant and Norplant II implants		Copper intrauterine devices	Levonorgestrel intrauterine devices	
	I	C	I	C	I	C	I	C	I	C	I	I	C
Cardiovascular disease													
Valvular heart disease													
a) Uncomplicated	2	2	2	2	1	1	1	1	1	1	1	1	1
b) Complicated (pulmonary hypertension, atrial fibrillation, history of subacute bacterial endocarditis)	4	4	4	4	1	1	1	1	1	1	2	2	2
Neurological conditions													
Headaches													
a) Non-migrainous (mild or severe)	1	2	1	2	1	1	1	1	1	1	1	1	1
b) Migraine													
i) without focal neurologic symptoms													
Age < 35	2	3	2	3	1	2	2	2	2	2	1	2	2
Age ≥ 35	3	4	3	4	1	2	2	2	2	2	1	2	2
ii) with focal neurologic symptoms (at any age)	4	4	4	4	2	3	2	3	2	2	1	2	3

I = initiation; **C** = continuation

Condition	Combined oral contraceptives	Combined injectable contraceptives	Progestogen-only pills	Depot-medroxy-progesterone acetate Norethisterone enanthate	Norplant and Norplant II implants	Copper intrauterine devices		Levonorgestrel intrauterine devices	
Neurological conditions									
Epilepsy	1	1	1	1	1	1		1	
Reproductive tract infections and disorders									
						I	**C**	**I**	**C**
Vaginal bleeding patterns									
a) Irregular pattern *without* heavy bleeding	1	1	2	2	2	1		1	1
b) Heavy or prolonged bleeding (includes regular and irregular patterns)	1	1	2	2	2	2		2	2
Unexplained vaginal bleeding (suspicious for serious condition)						**I**	**C**	**I**	**C**
Before evaluation	2	2	2	3	3	4	2	4	2
Endometriosis	1	1	1	1	1	2		1	

I = initiation; C = continuation

Condition	Combined oral contraceptives	Combined injectable contraceptives	Progestogen-only pills	Depot-medroxy-progesterone acetate Norethisterone enanthate	Norplant and Norplant II implants	Copper intrauterine devices	Levonorgestrel intrauterine devices
Reproductive tract infections and disorders							
Benign ovarian tumours (including cysts)	1	1	1	1	1	1	1
Severe dysmenorrhoea	1	1	1	1	1	2	1
Trophoblast disease a) Benign gestational trophoblastic disease	1	1	1	1	1	3	3
b) Malignant gestational trophic disease	1	1	1	1	1	4	4
Cervical ectropion	1	1	1	1	1	1	1
Cervical intraepithelial neoplasia (CIN)	2	2	1	2	2	1	2

Condition	Combined oral contraceptives	Combined injectable contraceptives	Progestogen-only pills	Depot-medroxy-progesterone acetate Norethisterone enanthate	Norplant and Norplant II implants	Copper intrauterine devices I	Copper C	Levonorgestrel intrauterine devices I	Levonorgestrel C
Reproductive tract infections and disorders									
Cervical cancer									
(awaiting treatment)	2	2	1	2	2	4	2	4	2
Breast disease									
a) Undiagnosed mass	2	2	2	2	2			2	2
b) Benign breast disease	1	1	1	1	1	1	1	1	1
c) Family history	1	1	1	1	1	1	1	1	1
d) Cancer									
i) current	4	4	4	4	4	1		4	4
ii) past and no evidence of current disease for 5 years	3	3	3	3	3	1		3	3
Endometrial cancer	1	1	1	1	1	4	2	4	2

I = initiation; C = continuation

Reproductive tract infections and disorders

Condition	Combined oral contraceptives	Combined injectable contraceptives	Progestogen-only pills	Depot-medroxyprogesterone acetate Norethisterone enanthate	Norplant and Norplant II implants	Copper intrauterine devices		Levonorgestrel intrauterine devices	
						I	**C**	**I**	**C**
Ovarian cancer	1	1	1	1	1	3	2	3	2
Uterine fibroids									
a) Without distortion of the uterine cavity	1	1	1	1	1	1	1	1	1
b) With distortion of the uterine cavity	1	1	1	1	1	4	4	4	4
Pelvic inflammatory disease (PID)						**I**	**C**	**I**	**C**
a) Past PID (assuming no current risk factor of STIs)									
i) with subsequent pregnancy	1	1	1	1	1	1	1	1	1
ii) without subsequent pregnancy	1	1	1	1	1	2	2	2	2
b) PID-current or within the last 3 months	1	1	1	1	1	4	2	4	2

I = initiation; **C** = continuation

Condition	Combined oral contraceptives	Combined injectable contraceptives	Progestogen-only pills	Depot-medroxy-progesterone acetate Norethisterone enanthate	Norplant and Norplant II implants	Copper intrauterine devices	Levonorgestrel intrauterine devices
Reproductive tract infections and disorders							
STIs[3]							
a) Current or within 3 months (including purulent cervicitis)	1	1	1	1	1	4	4
b) Vaginitis without purulent cervicitis	1	1	1	1	1	2	2
c) Increased risk of STIs (e.g. multiple partners or partner who has had multiple partners)	1	1	1	1	1	3	3
HIV/AIDS[3]							
High risk of HIV	1	1	1	1	1	3	3
HIV-positive	1	1	1	1	1	3	3
AIDS	1	1	1	1	1	3	3

[3]Barrier methods, especially condoms, are always recommended for prevention of sexually transmitted infections (STIs)/HIV/PID

Condition	Combined oral contraceptives	Combined injectable contraceptives	Progestogen-only pills	Depot-medroxy-progesterone acetate Norethisterone enanthate	Norplant and Norplant II implants	Copper intrauterine devices		Levonorgestrel intrauterine devices	
Other infections									
Schistosomiasis									
a) Uncomplicated	1	1	1	1	1	1		1	
b) Liver fibrosis	1	1	1	1	1	1		1	
Tuberculosis						I	C	I	C
a) Non-pelvic	1	1	1	1	1	1	1	1	1
b) Known pelvic	1	1	1	1	1	4	3	4	3
Malaria	1	1	1	1	1	1		1	

I = initiation; **C** = continuation

Condition	Combined oral contraceptives	Combined injectable contraceptives	Progestogen-only pills	Depot-medroxy-progesterone acetate Norethisterone enanthate	Norplant and Norplant II implants	Copper intrauterine devices	Levonorgestrel intrauterine devices
Endocrine conditions							
Diabetes							
a) History of gestational diabetes	1	1	1	1	1	1	1
b) Non-vascular disease							
) non-insulin dependent	2	2	2	2	2	1	2
ii) insulin dependent	2	2	2	2	2	1	2
c) Nephropathy/retinopathy/neuropathy	3/4	3/4	2	3	2	1	2
d) Other vascular disease or diabetes of > 20 years' duration	3/4	3/4	2	3	2	1	2
Thyroid							
a) Simple goitre	1	1	1	1	1	1	1
b) Hyperthyroid	1	1	1	1	1	1	1
c) Hypothyroid	1	1	1	1	1	1	1

Condition	Combined oral contraceptives	Combined injectable contraceptives	Progestogen-only pills	Depot-medroxyprogesterone acetate Norethisterone enanthate	Norplant and Norplant II implants	Copper intrauterine devices	Levonorgestrel intrauterine devices
Gastrointestinal conditions							
Gall bladder disease							
a) Symptomatic							
i) treated by cholecystectomy	2	2	2	2	2	1	2
ii) medically treated	3	2	2	2	2	1	2
iii) current	3	2	2	2	2	1	2
b) Asymptomatic	2	2	2	2	2	1	2
History of cholestasis							
a) Pregnancy-related	2	2	1	1	1	1	1
b) Past COC-related	3	2	2	2	2	1	2
Viral hepatitis							
a) Active	4	3/4	3	3	3	1	3
b) Carrier	1	1	1	1	1	1	1
Cirrhosis							
a) Mild (compensated)	3	2	2	2	2	1	3
b) Severe (decompensated)	4	3	3	3	3	1	3

Condition	Combined oral contraceptives	Combined injectable contraceptives	Progestogen-only pills	Depot-medroxyprogesterone acetate Norethisterone enanthate	Norplant and Norplant II implants	Copper intrauterine devices	Levonorgestrel intrauterine devices
Gastrointestinal conditions							
Liver tumours							
a) Benign (adenoma)	4	3	3	3	3	1	3
b) Malignant (hepatoma)	4	3/4	3	3	3	1	3
Anaemias							
Thalassaemia	1	1	1	1	1	2	1
Sickle cell disease	2	2	1	1	1	2	1
Iron-deficiency anaemia	1	1	1	1	1	2	1

Condition	Combined oral contraceptives	Combined injectable contraceptives	Progestogen-only pills	Depot-medroxy-progesterone acetate Norethisterone enanthate	Norplant and Norplant II implants	Copper intrauterine devices	Levonorgestrel intrauterine devices
Drug interactions							
Commonly used drugs that affect liver enzymes							
a) Certain antibiotics (rifampicin and griseofulvin)	3	3	3	2	3	1	1
b) Certain anticonvulsants (phenytoin, carbamazepine, barbiturates, primidone)	3	3	3	2	3	1	1
Other antibiotics (excluding rifampicin and griseofulvin)	1	1	1	1	1	1	1

Appendix 2 – Contraceptives

A. Intrauterine devices and depot contraceptives

Intrauterine devices

Name	Features	Specific use
Multiload Cu 250	Copper wire on plastic stem with flexible U-shaped side-arms and monofilament thread	Uterine length 6–9cm; replace every 3 years
Multiload Cu 250 short	As Multiload Cu 250	Uterine length 5–7 cm; replace every 3 years
Multiload Cu 375	As Multiload Cu 250	Uterine length 6–9 cm; replace every 5 years
Multi-safe 375	Copper wire on plastic stem with flexible U-shaped side-arms and monofilament thread	Replace after 5 years
Nova-T 380	Copper wire with silver core on T-shaped carrier with monofilament thread	Uterine length 6.5–9 cm; replace every 5 years
Flexi-T 300	Copper wire on a T-shaped carrier with monofilament thread	Uterine length > 5 cm; replace every 5 years
GyneFix	Frameless, flexible device with six copper tubes on knotted suture thread implanted in myometrium	Inserted by trained doctor only; replace after 5 years
T-Safe CU 380A	T-shaped plastic carrier with copper wire on vertical stem and copper sleeves on horizontal arms	Uterine length 6.5–9 cm; replace after 8–10 years

Name	Features	Specific use
A. Intrauterine devices and depot contraceptives		
Intrauterine systems		
Mirena	T-shaped intrauterine system containing 52 mg levonorgestrel	Replace after 5 years
Injectables		
DepoProvera	Medroxyprogesterone acetate 150 mg/ml in prefilled syringe/vials	150 mg by intramuscular injection every 12 weeks
Noristerat	Norethisterone enanthate 200 mg in 1-ml ampoule	Short-term use; intramuscular injection of 200 mg every 8 weeks
Implant		
Implanon	Etonogestrel 68 mg, subdermal implant	Replace within 3 years
Transdermal patch		
Ortho Evra	Continuous daily release of ethinyloestradiol 20 µg/norelgestromin 150 µg	Replace after 7 days

Formulation	Name	Oestrogen dose (μg)	Progestogen dose (mg)
B. Oral contraceptives			
Combined pills			
Monophasic			
Ethinyloestradiol/levonorgestrel	Microgynon 30/Microgynon 30 ED	30	0.15
	Ovranette	30	0.15
	Eugynon 30	30	0.25
	Ovran 30	30	0.25
Ethinyloestradiol/norethisterone type	Loestrin 20	20	1
	Loestrin 30	30	1.5
	Brevinor	35	0.5
	Ovysmen	35	0.5
	Norimin	35	1
Ethinyloestradiol/desogestrel	Mercilon	20	0.15
	Marvelon	30	0.15
Ethinyloestradiol/ gestodene	Femodene/Femodene ED	30	0.075
	Minulet	30	0.075
	Femodette	20	0.075
Ethinyloestradiol/ norgestimate	Cilest	35	0.25
Mestranol/ norethisterone	Norinyl-1	50	1

Formulation	Name	Oestrogen dose (μg)	Progestogen dose (mg)
B. Oral contraceptives			
Combined pills			
Biphasic and triphasic pills			
Ethinyloestradiol/ levonorgestrel	Logynon/Logynon ED	30	0.05 (six tablets)
		40	0.075 (five tablets)
		30	0.125 (10 tablets)
	Triordiol	30	0.05 (six tablets)
		40	0.075 (five tablets)
		30	0.125 (10 tablets)
Ethinyloestradiol/norethisterone	BiNovum	35	0.5 (seven tablets)
		35	1 (14 tablets)
	Synphase	35	0.5 (seven tablets)
		35	1 (nine tablets)
		35	0.5 (five tablets)
	TriNovum	35	0.5 (seven tablets)
		35	0.75 (seven tablets)
		35	1 (seven tablets)
Ethinylestradiol/ gestodene	Tri-Minulet	30	0.05 (six tablets)
		40	0.07 (five tablets)
		30	0.1 (10 tablets)
	Triadene	30	0.05 (six tablets)
		40	0.07 (five tablets)
		30	0.1 (10 tablets)

Formulation	Name	Oestrogen dose (µg)	Progestogen dose (mg)
B. Oral contraceptives			
Combined pills			
Biphasic and triphasic pills			
Ethinyloestradiol/drosperinone	Yasmin	30	3.00
Progestogen-only pills			
Levonorgestrel	Microval	–	0.03
	Norgeston	–	0.03
Norgestrel	Neogest	–	0.075
Norethisterone type	Micronor	–	0.35
	Noriday	–	0.35
	Femulen	–	0.5
Desogestrel	Cerazette	–	0.75

Appendix 3 – Useful websites

General

http://www.who.int/reproductive-health
WHO medical eligibility criteria and selected practice recommendations

http://www.ffprhc.org.uk
UK Faculty of Family Planning guidelines, electronic journal

http://www.hilo.nhs.uk
Free full text journals for NHS employees

http://www.fpa.org.uk
UK Family Planning Association's contraception user website; has Family Planning Association leaflets

http://www.fertilityuk.org
Fertility awareness/natural family planning material and contacts

http://www.rcog.org.uk
UK Royal College of Obstetricians and Gynaecologists – RCOG evidence-based guidelines

http://www.acog.com
The American College of Obstetricians and Gynecologists

**http://www.cdc.gov and
www.cdc.gov/publications.htm**
US Centers for Disease Control and Prevention – prevention guidelines

http://www.fda.gov
US Food and Drug Administration

http://www.nih.gov
US National Institutes of Health – free biomedical research centres; wide medical information resource

http://www.ppfa.org/pppfa/index.html
Planned Parenthood Federation of America

http://www.fhi.org
Reproductive and sexual health website of Family Health International research organization

http://www.agi-usa.org
Allan Guttmacher Institute

http://www.contraception—esc.com
European Society of Contraception

http://www.ippf.org
International Planned Parenthood Federation

Health education websites
http://www.interactworldwide.org
Global safer sex education resource

http://www.playingsafely.co.uk
A fun sexual health site

http://contraceptiononlline.org
Online resource – Baylor College of Medicine, supported by Wyeth

http://www.contraceptioneducation.co.uk
Sexual health for young people

AIDS websites

http://www.unaids.org
AIDS resource from UN programme on HIV/AIDS

http://www.ama-assn.org and
http://www.pubs.ama-assn.org
JAMA HIV/AIDS information

http://www.positive.org
Coalition for Positive Sexuality and Just Say Yes

http://www.epibiostat.ucsf.edu/capsweb
The Center for AIDS Prevention Studies (CAPS)

http://www.safersex.org
The Safer Sex site

Cancer websites

http://www.nbcc.org.au
The breast cancer evidence based information

http://www.cancernet.nci.nih.gov
CancerNet

http://www.nci.nih.gov
National Cancer Institute

Emergency contraception websites

http://www.cecinfo.org
The Consortium for Emergency Contraception (USA)

http://ec.princeton.edu/
Princeton University's emergency contraception website

http://www.who.int/reproductive-health/
family_planning/methods.html
WHO emergency contraception database

Evidence-based medicine websites/clinical information websites

http://www.cochrane.org

http://www.unaids.org

http://www.ncbi.nlm.nih.gov/pubmed

http://www.prodigy.nhs.uk

http://www.clinicalevidence.com

http://nelh.nhs.uk
National Electronic Library for Health

Index

Note: Abbreviations: as listed on page x. Page numbers followed by 'f' indicate figures; page numbers followed by 't' indicate tables.